Food Safety Culture

Food Microbiology and Food Safety Series

Food Microbiology and Food Safety publishes valuable, practical, and timely resources for professionals and researchers working on microbiological topics associated with foods, as well as food safety issues and problems.

Series Editor

Michael P. Doyle, *Regents Professor and Director of the Center for Food Safety, University of Georgia, Griffith, GA, USA*

Editorial Board

Francis F. Busta, *Director, National Center for Food Protection and Defense, University of Minnesota, Minneapolis, MN, USA*
Bruce R. Cords, *Vice President, Environment, Food Safety & Public Health, Ecolab Inc., St. Paul, MN, USA*
Catherine W. Donnelly, *Professor of Nutrition and Food Science, University of Vermont, Burlington, VT, USA*
Paul A. Hall, *President, AIV Microbiology and Food Safety Consultants, LLC, Hawthorn Woods, IL, USA*
Ailsa D. Hocking, *Chief Research Scientist, CSIRO—Food Science Australia, North Ryde, Australia*
Thomas J. Montville, *Professor of Food Microbiology, Rutgers University, New Brunswick, NJ, USA*
R. Bruce Tompkin, *Formerly Vice President-Product Safety, ConAgra Refrigerated Prepared Foods, Downers Grove, IL, USA*

Titles

Effective Risk Communication: A Message-Centered Approach, Timothy L. Sellnow, Robert R. Ulmer, Matthew W. Seeger, Robert S. Littlefield (Eds.) (2009)
Food Safety Culture, Frank Yiannas (2008)
Molecular Techniques in the Microbial Ecology of Fermented Foods, Luca Cocolin and Danilo Ercolini (Eds.) (2008)
Viruses in Foods, Sagar M. Goyal (Ed.) (2006)
Foodborne Parasites, Ynes R. Ortega (Ed.) (2006)
PCR Methods in Foods, John Maurer (Ed.) (2006)

Frank Yiannas

Food Safety Culture

Creating a Behavior-Based Food Safety Management System

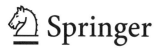

Frank Yiannas
Bentonville, Arkansas
USA
foodsafetyculture@msn.com

ISBN: 978-0-387-72866-7   e-ISBN: 978-0-387-72867-4
DOI 10.1007/978-0-387-72867-4

Library of Congress Control Number: 2008935903

© 2009 Springer Science+Business Media, LLC
All rights reserved. This work may not be translated or copied in whole or in part without the written permission of the publisher (Springer Science+Business Media, LLC, 233 Spring Street, New York, NY 10013, USA), except for brief excerpts in connection with reviews or scholarly analysis. Use in connection with any form of information storage and retrieval, electronic adaptation, computer software, or by similar or dissimilar methodology now known or hereafter developed is forbidden. The use in this publication of trade names, trademarks, service marks, and similar terms, even if they are not identified as such, is not to be taken as an expression of opinion as to whether or not they are subject to proprietary rights.

Printed on acid-free paper

springer.com

This book is dedicated to my parents, Haralambos and Daisy Yiannas, for teaching me through their example and not just words, the importance of a strong work ethic and always searching for a better way.

Contents

1	**Looking Back to Shape the Future**...........................	1
	History of Food Production...............................	1
	Emergence of Retail Food Establishments...................	3
	Foodborne Disease.....................................	4
	Retail Food Safety.....................................	6
	Reducing Risk Early in the Food Production Chain..........	6
	Changing Behavior................................	8
	Key Points...	9
2	**Why the Focus on Culture?**................................	11
	What Is Culture?......................................	11
	Why Is Culture Important?...............................	12
	Who Creates Culture?...................................	13
	How Is Culture Created?.................................	14
	The Foundation.......................................	15
	Core Elements..	15
	Leadership at the Top..............................	16
	Confidence in the Part of All Employees....................	16
	Clear Management Visibility and Leadership.................	16
	Accountability at All Levels........................	17
	Sharing of Knowledge and Information.....................	17
	Best Practices...	17
	Key Points...	18
3	**A Systems-Based Approach to Food Safety**......................	21
	What Is a System?.....................................	22
	Systems Thinking......................................	22
	Behavior Change Theories and Models........................	23
	Behavioral Theory................................	23
	Social Cognitive Theory................................	23
	Health Belief Model.................................	24
	Theory of Reasoned Action...........................	24

       Transtheoretical Model.................................. 24
       Social Marketing....................................... 25
   Environmental or Physical Factors........................... 25
   A Behavior-Based Systems Continuous Improvement Model..... 27
   Key Points.. 28

4 Creating Food Safety Performance Expectations................. 29
   Getting Employees to Do What They Are Supposed to Do....... 29
   Expect More than Efficiency............................... 30
   Expect a Proper Food Safety Attitude....................... 31
   Be Specific – Not Generic................................. 31
   Start with the Food Code................................. 32
   Develop Risk-Based Expectations.......................... 32
   Beyond Regulatory Compliance............................ 34
   Write Them All Down.................................... 35
   Key Points.. 36

5 Educating and Training to Influence Behavior.................. 39
   Education Versus Training................................ 40
   Why Educate and Train?.................................. 41
   Focus on Changing Behavior.............................. 42
   Make It Risk-Based..................................... 44
   Value and Respect Diversity.............................. 44
   Keep It Simple and User Friendly......................... 45
   Key Points.. 46

6 Communicating Food Safety Effectively....................... 49
   The Importance of Communication......................... 49
   Use a Variety of Mediums................................ 50
   Posters, Symbols, and Slogans............................ 51
   Use More than Words.................................... 51
   Have Conversations..................................... 52
   Ask Questions.. 54
   Key Points.. 55

7 Developing Food Safety Goals and Measurements............... 57
   The Importance of Food Safety Goal Setting................. 57
   Establishing Effective Food Safety Goals................... 58
   Why Measure Food Safety?............................... 59
   What Should You Measure?.............................. 61
   Lagging Versus Leading Indicators of Food Safety............ 62
   Key Points.. 65

8	**Using Consequences to Increase or Decrease Behaviors**	67
	Determine the Cause of Performance Problems	68
	Creating Consequences for Food Safety	69
	Positive Consequences	70
	Negative Consequences	73
	Key Points	74
9	**Tying It All Together – Behavior-Based Food Safety Management** . .	77
	Management or Leadership?	77
	Traditional Food Safety Management Versus Behavior-Based Food Safety Management	78
10	**Unwrapping – Thoughts on the Future of Food Safety**	83
	The Way Forward?	83
	Making Significant Leaps	84
	The Future	85
References		87
Index		91

Introduction

It has been said, *what we know and what we believe is of little consequence. It is what we do that is important.* When it comes to food safety, this point is certainly true.

The main reason I decided to write this book is simple. It's because I wish I could have known 20 years ago (when I started my career in food safety) what I know now. The concepts I will share with you in this book are not generally taught in food science curriculums. They are not something you generally hear about in food safety seminars or at food safety conferences. To my knowledge, there is not much documented in the food safety literature about this topic.

The concepts you'll read about in this book are simple. Many are age-old principles about human behavior. Others are more recent concepts developed through the study of human behavior, group dynamics, and organizational culture. Many of the ideas may be considered simple. They are so simple that they are powerful. In fact, one of the most common compliments I receive is that the ideas presented in this text are simple, but they are rarely assembled together in this manner and they are rarely used in the context of improved food safety performance.

In the field of food safety today, there is much documented about specific microbes, time/temperature processes, post-process contamination, and HACCP – things often called the hard sciences. There is not much published or discussed related to human behavior and culture – often referred to as the "soft stuff."

However, if you look at foodborne disease trends over the past few decades, it's clear to me that the soft stuff is still the hard stuff. We won't make dramatic improvements in reducing the global burden of foodborne disease, especially in certain parts of the food system and world, until we get much better at influencing and changing human behavior (the soft stuff).

Despite the fact that thousands of employees have been trained in food safety around the world, millions have been spent globally on food safety research, and countless inspections and tests have been performed at home and abroad, food safety remains a significant public health challenge. Why is that? The answer to this question reminds me of a quote by Elliot M. Estes, who said, *"If something has been done a particular way for 15 or 20 years, it's a pretty good* sign, in these changing times, that it is being done the wrong way." To improve food safety, we have to realize that it's more than just food science; it's the behavioral sciences too.

Think about it. If you're trying to improve the food safety performance of an organization, industry, or region of the world, what you're really trying to do is change peoples' behaviors. *Simply put, food safety equals behavior*. This is the fundamental premise that this entire book is based upon.

Before you read this book, let me share what it is intended to be and what it is not.

This book is intended to be:

- An introductory textbook on the topic of behavior-based food safety
- An easy to use, quick reference guide on key concepts of a behavior-based food safety management system
- Primarily for food safety professionals

This book is not intended to be:

- A highly technical reference manual
- A step by step instructions manual
- The only resource for those with an interest in the behavioral sciences or behavior-based food safety

This book is devoted to providing you with new ideas and concepts that have not been thoroughly reviewed, researched, and discussed in the field of food safety. It is my wish that by simply reading this book, you pick up a few ideas, tips, or approaches that can help you further improve future food safety performance within your organization or area of responsibility. By sharing and learning from each other as professionals, we can make a difference, advance food safety worldwide, and improve the quality of life for consumers all over the world.

Frank

If you have any questions, comments, or suggestions, I would love to hear from you. You can e-mail me at foodsafetyculture@msn.com Thanks for reading.

Chapter 1
Looking Back to Shape the Future

> *A prescription without diagnosis is malpractice.*
> Socrates (469 BC–399 BC)

Food safety awareness is at an all-time high; new and emerging threats to the food supply are being recognized; and consumers are eating more and more meals prepared outside of the home. Accordingly, retail and foodservice establishments, as well as food producers at all levels of the food production chain, have a growing responsibility to ensure that proper food safety and sanitation practices are followed, thereby safeguarding the health of their customers.

Achieving food safety success in this changing environment often requires going beyond traditional training, testing, and inspectional approaches to managing risks. It requires a better understanding of organizational culture and the human dimensions of food safety.

To improve the food safety performance of a retail or foodservice establishment, an organization with thousands of employees, or a local community, you must change the way people do things. You must change their behavior. In fact, simply put, often times food safety equals behavior (Fig. 1.1).

When viewed from this perspective, one of the most common contributing causes of foodborne disease is unsafe human behavior. Thus, to improve food safety, we need to better integrate the food sciences with the behavioral sciences and use a systems-based approach to managing food safety risk.

This book is devoted to providing new ideas and approaches that can help you further improve the future food safety performance within your organization or area of responsibility. But in order to shape the future of food safety, it's important to understand and learn from the past.

History of Food Production

Throughout human history, our existence has been dependant on food. However, how we get our food and produce our food has changed dramatically over the years. Our concern and knowledge about foodborne disease has changed dramatically too.

Archaeologists believe that in the early days of human existence, humans primarily hunted and gathered their food. Small social and family groups formed for survival and to hunt, fish, and gather food. After years of small

Fig. 1.1 Food safety equation

Food Safety = Behavior

groups moving from one place to another in search of food, the way humans gathered food started to change. In certain parts of the world more favorable for gathering and cultivating food, humans began to learn how to cultivate crops and domesticate animals and they started to form small villages. Early farming practices became established, which allowed groups of people to live in the same geographic region for longer periods of time.

Over many hundreds of years and at the dawn of the 20th century, a significant percentage of the world's population was still directly involved in farming or agriculture. Many individuals and families would still grow and raise their own food, but they were able to produce more crops and raise more animals on a limited area of land than ever before and, thereby, feed a larger and growing population. Advancements in agriculture are believed to have been one of the major driving forces in the formation of cities and many components that define modern civilization. Increased food production led to decreases in food prices for individuals living in urban areas. With increased food production, individuals were no longer required to produce their own food. They could pursue other professions or labor specialties. This also led to more leisure time for individuals to pursue other interests and activities.

Today, the way we get our food from farm to fork, the food system, has evolved into an increasingly complex network interdependent on many businesses, sectors, and individuals. The United States Department of Agriculture, Economic Research Service (2006) defines the term "food system" as "a complex network of farmers and the industries that link to them. Those links include makers of farm equipment and chemicals as well as firms that provide services to agribusinesses, such as providers of transportation and financial services. The system also includes the food marketing industries that link farms to consumers and which include food and fiber processors, wholesalers, retailers, and foodservice establishments."

This modern food system is interdependent on various elements including technology for production and processing, various forms of transportation for the movement of food, integrated information management for supply chain logistics and inventory control, marketing for reaching consumers, and much more. When it comes to food safety, within this complex system there are numerous critical control points needed to manage food safety risk, often times not integrated as well as they should be.

Adding to the complexity of the food system is the fact that the food supply is becoming more global. As our global community expands, the business of moving food from the farm to the dinner table has become increasingly complex. Food is being distributed further than ever before, sometimes from one distant country to another, and foodborne disease outbreaks have the growing potential of being widespread. This trend is occurring worldwide.

Emergence of Retail Food Establishments

In today's complex food system, consumers are becoming increasingly removed from most aspects of food production. Retail food establishments, in this book broadly defined to include both supermarkets and foodservice establishments, have emerged as the main point where consumers now get their food.

Supermarkets allow consumers to buy thousands of different types of food products, fresh and processed, all in one convenient location with a continuous, year-round supply. Both supermarkets and foodservice establishments also allow consumers to buy already prepared food and meals.

It has been estimated that in an average life, a person will eat more than 75,000 meals (Cliver, 1990). Just a few decades ago, most of those meals were prepared inside the home. As more and more households began to be comprised of dual working spouses, it has become increasingly difficult to find time to prepare food in today's busy society (Gallup, 1999).

Today, consumers are eating more and more of those meals outside of the home On a typical day, 44% of adults in the United States eat at a restaurant (NRA, 2001). As shown in Fig. 1.2, according to Ebbin (2001), approximately 46% of the U.S. food dollar is now spent on restaurant meals. And more than 54 billion meals are served at 844,000 commercial food establishments in the United States annually (NRA, 2001).

The restaurant industry is now reported to be the largest private-sector employer in the United States providing jobs for 12.5 million employees (NRA, 2006). And this number is expected to grow. As illustrated in Fig. 1.3, it's reported that on average, one out of every four restaurant employees in the United States does not speak English at home (NRA, 2006). In some states with large Hispanic populations, these numbers can be higher. With such a large and diverse workforce with high turnover rates, recruitment, retention, and training strategies are critically important.

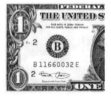 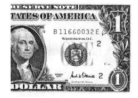

Fig. 1.2 U.S. food dollar spent (2002)

**$414 Billion (46%)
Food Away From Home**

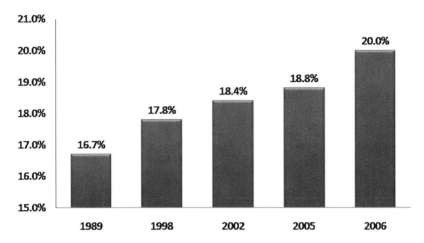

Fig. 1.3 Estimated percentage of restaurant employees speaking a language other than English at home

Although there is no question that the emergence of retail food establishments as a key component of today's food system has provided consumers with a more diverse food supply and convenient source of prepared, economical, and ready-to-eat meals, these trends have resulted in both benefits and additional risks. With an increasing number of meals now being consumed outside of the home in a record number of retail establishments with an incredibly large workforce with high turnover and foods sourced from all over the world, retail food establishments have a challenging responsibility to source safe food products and ingredients and to prepare food safely, thereby, safeguarding the health of their customers.

Foodborne Disease

Although we do not know with certainty the true incidence of foodborne disease, as shown in Fig. 1.4, in the United States alone, the Centers for Disease Control and Prevention estimates that each year diseases caused by food may result in 325,000 serious illnesses resulting in hospitalizations, 76 million cases of gastrointestinal illnesses, and up to 5,000 deaths (Mead, Slutsker, & Dietz et al., 1999).

Of a mean 550 foodborne disease outbreaks reported to the Centers for Disease Control and Prevention each year from 1993 through 1997 (Fig. 1.5), a large percentage, over 40%, were linked to commercial foodservice establishments (Olsen, MacKinon, Goulding, Bean, & Slutsker, 2000). Statistics such as this are often used to claim that retail food establishments are responsible for a large percentage of foodborne disease outbreaks in the United States.

Fig. 1.4 Estimate of foodborne disease in the United States per year

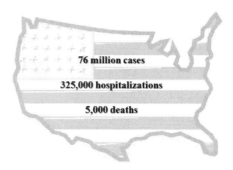

However, these data must be interpreted with caution. The association between two events is not the same as cause and effect. Epidemiological patterns consist of patterns between time, place, and persons. It is this triad that has historically allowed more foodborne illnesses involving foodservice establishments and institutions to be recognized.

With improved foodborne surveillance, better detection tools, and shifts in the responsibility for food safety, these trends may change. More and more, public health officials are now detecting seemingly unrelated illnesses to a common food source and, often times, foodservice establishments are not responsible.

Also, it must be recognized that the place where the food was eaten is not necessarily the same as or related to the point at which the food was contaminated or where the microbiological agent survived processing or multiplied to levels sufficient to cause illness. When conducting foodborne investigations, data on where the contamination occurred and where the food was mishandled should also be collected, which may provide more useful information.

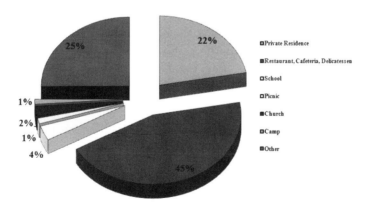

Fig. 1.5 Number of reported foodborne outbreaks in the United States by place (CDC, 1993–1997) (*See* Color Insert)

Nevertheless, despite the inability to draw absolute conclusions from foodborne disease data, preventing restaurant-associated foodborne disease outbreaks remains an important public health priority and a growing challenge.

Retail Food Safety

Historically, the two primary methods used to reduce the risk of foodborne disease in retail establishments have been regulatory inspections and training. In the United States, retail food establishments are regularly inspected by local, county, or state health departments. In some parts of the country, restaurant inspection reports and scores are becoming increasingly accessible to the public and the local media through the Internet.

But are retail food inspections really effective at reducing the risk of foodborne disease? Several studies documented in the scientific literature, such as those by Jones, Pavlin, LaFleur, Ingram, and Schaffner (2004) and Mullen, Cowden, Cowden, and Wong (2002), have suggested that there is no correlation between retail food safety inspection scores and the likelihood that an establishment might be involved in an outbreak. Moreover, results from the last two FDA baseline surveys (FDA Retail Food Program Steering Committee, 2000) suggest that despite thousands of health department inspections and thousands of employees trained in food safety, inspection outcomes of retail food establishments in the United States are not significantly improving over time (FDA National Retail Food Team, 2004).

This quote by Chris Griffith from the University of Wales Institute summarizes this point quite well. He said, "In spite of over 100 years of research and millions of dollars spent, food safety remains a worldwide public health issue."

If thousands of inspections of retail food establishments are being conducted, millions of dollars are being spent on food safety research, and thousands of retail food employees are being trained in food safety across the country, then why haven't we seen the types of dramatic reductions in retail-associated foodborne disease that many of us would like to? Although there are probably several valid reasons, let me summarize two very important points. One, it's important that we realize that some retail food safety risk is best controlled very early in the food production chain, not in the retail establishment. And two, often times, to improve food safety at the retail level, we have to change the way people do things. We must change their behavior.

Reducing Risk Early in the Food Production Chain

As we look for strategies to reduce foodborne risks in retail establishments, it's important to realize that for many years the methods we have been using have

1 Looking Back to Shape the Future

not produced the desired dramatic reductions in overall foodborne disease. Therefore, in order to dramatically reduce risk, future prevention strategies must focus on eliminating the presence of pathogenic organisms on raw and processed products before they enter retail and foodservice establishments, rather than eliminating them at the restaurant or preventing their growth.

With this thought in mind, let me introduce you to a new term I've been using that is called strategic control points (SCP). We must realize that some risk is best controlled very early in the food production chain and that not all critical control points (CCP) are equal. Some are clearly more effective or strategic than others. For a visual model, see Fig. 1.6.

Let me explain what I mean. For example, if you look at FoodNet data (CDC, 2007), *Campylobacter* is one of the most common causes of bacterial foodborne disease in this country. And it is often associated with mishandled poultry products. If we truly want to reduce the incidence of *Campylobacter* among the U.S. population, let us focus on developing a very effective Strategic Control Point. If we can reduce rates of contamination of *Campylobacter* early in the food production chain, I am quite confident that the number of human cases of *Campylobacter* will dramatically drop. But if we continue to rely on the final cook, whether it be in a restaurant or in a home, our risk reduction benefits will be less noticeable.

Remember, there is a shared responsibility for food safety at the retail level. The days where the buck stops with the cook or the restaurant are, in my opinion, close to being behind us. The responsibility lies along the entire food

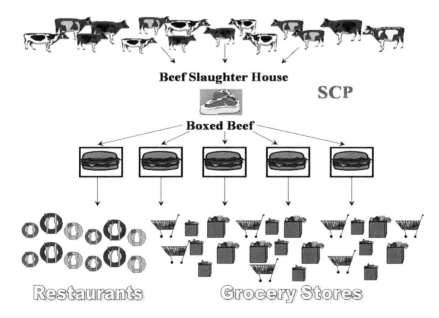

Fig. 1.6 Visual model of a strategic control point (SCP)

production chain. Retail establishments must and will continue to do their part, but we need to get better as an industry in reducing food safety risk very early in the food production chain.

Changing Behavior

Although the first and very crucial step to addressing food safety risk at the retail level is to manage food safety risk very early in the food production chain, once food enters the retail food establishment, it must be stored and prepared safely by retail employees.

As illustrated in Fig. 1.7, some of the more common contributing factors of foodborne outbreaks reported to the Centers for Disease and Prevention include improper holding temperatures, inadequate cooking, contaminated equipment, and poor personal hygiene (Olsen et al., 2000). But upon a closer examination of these contributing factors, instead of looking at them as technical or epidemiological classifications, I see and visualize something very different. For example, when I think of the contributing factor of undercooked food, I can visualize someone at a grill, undercooking a beef pattie. In other words, I see a behavior. How about the contributing factor of contaminated equipment? When I think about this contributing factor, I can imagine someone using a cutting board to cut raw meat and then using that same cutting board, without adequately washing and sanitizing it in between uses, to cut a salad, a ready-to-eat produce item. Again, I see a behavior. How about the contributing factor of poor personal hygiene? Rather than thinking about this as a technical classification, I can see persons failing to wash their hands when they're

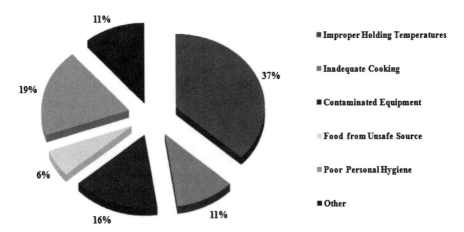

Fig. 1.7 Number of reported foodborne outbreaks in the United States by contributing factor (CDC, 1993–1997) (*See* Color Insert)

supposed to or employees coming to work when they're ill. I see a behavior. The bottom line is that often times, food safety equals behavior.

Historically, the two primary methods used to reduce the risk of foodborne disease in retail establishments have been regulatory inspections and training. It's important that we realize that inspections and training, although two very important methods to improving retail food safety, are not the first steps in this process, nor are they the only steps in this process – and they are certainly not enough. Achieving food safety success in retail establishments, as well as other levels of the food supply chain, requires going beyond traditional training, testing, and inspectional approaches to managing risks. It requires a better understanding of organizational culture and the human dimensions of food safety. To improve the food safety performance of a retail or foodservice establishment, an organization with thousands of employees, or a local community, you must change the way people do things. You must change their behavior.

Achieving food safety success often requires more than a thorough understanding of the food sciences. It requires better integration of the food sciences with the behavioral sciences to create a behavior-based food safety management system or food safety culture – not just a food safety program.

For the remainder of this book, we will focus on this unique aspect of food safety – behavior and culture.

Key Points

- Food safety awareness is at an all-time high; new and emerging threats to the food supply are being recognized; and consumers are eating more and more meals prepared outside of the home.
- How we get our food and how we produce our food have changed dramatically over the years.
- Retail food establishments have emerged as the main point where consumers now get their food.
- Although there is no question that the emergence of retail food establishments as a key component of today's food system has provided consumers with a more diverse food supply and convenient source of prepared, economical, and ready-to-eat meals, these trends have resulted in both benefits and additional risks.
- Historically, the two primary methods used to reduce the risk of foodborne disease in retail establishments have been regulatory inspections and training.
- Despite thousands of inspections of retail food establishments being conducted and thousands of retail food employees being trained, we have not seen the types of dramatic reductions in retail-associated foodborne disease that many of us would like to.

- Some retail food safety risk is best controlled very early in the food production chain, not in the retail establishment, through the creation of strategic control points (SCPs).
- To improve food safety at the retail level, we have to change the way people do things. We must change their behavior.
- Better integration of the food sciences with the behavioral sciences is needed to create a *behavior-based food safety management system*.

Chapter 2
Why the Focus on Culture?

> *Every man's ability may be strengthened or increased by culture.*
> Sir John Abbott, 3rd Prime Minster of Canada (1821–1893)

If your organization's goal is to create a bigger or better food safety program, then I suggest that although you may be well intentioned, you might be missing the mark? Your goal should be to create a food safety culture – not a food safety program (Fig. 2.1). There is a big difference between the two.

Culture is one of those terms getting used often in today's society, maybe even overused. So what does it really mean? The words we choose and how we use them are important. They're more important than we sometimes realize. They're the foundation of effective communication. So let's take a moment to review the word culture.

What Is Culture?

As a food scientist, culture may be one of those terms that seems a little fuzzy or abstract. It's hard for us to wrap our arms around it. We feel much more comfortable talking about specific microbes, pH, water activity, and temperature. We consider these the hard science. We feel less comfortable talking about terms related to human behavior such as culture – often called the "soft stuff." To make this point, let's pretend you were to ask 10 different food scientists to define culture for you. What do you think their answers would be? It's very likely that you would get 10 different answers. But if you were to ask these same 10 individuals to define pH or water activity, I suspect their answers would be much more similar.

If you look at foodborne disease trends over the past few decades, it's clear to me that the soft stuff is still the hard stuff. We won't make dramatic improvements in reducing the global burden of foodborne disease, especially in certain parts of the food system and world, until we get much better at influencing and changing human behavior (the soft stuff).

So what is culture? Well, one of the best definitions that I've come across (Coreil, Bryant, and Henderson, 2001) states "Culture is patterned ways of thought and behavior that characterize a social group, which can be learned through socialization processes and persist through time." Accordingly, from

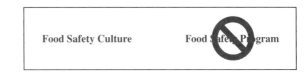

Fig. 2.1 Food safety culture – not a food safety program

our perspective, a food safety culture can then be viewed as how and what the employees in a company or organization think about food safety. It's the food safety behaviors that they routinely practice and demonstrate. According to this definition, employees will learn these thoughts and behaviors by simply becoming part of the company or organizational group. Furthermore, these thoughts or behaviors will permeate throughout the entire organization. And if you truly create a food safety culture, these thoughts and behaviors will be sustained over time as opposed to being the "program of the month" or this year's focus.

A more technical definition by the Health and Safety Commission (1993) states, "The safety culture of an organization is the product of the individual and group values, attitudes, competencies and patterns of behavior that determine the commitment to, and the style and proficiency of, an organization's health and safety programs. Organizations with a positive safety culture are characterized by communications founded on mutual trust, by shared perceptions of the importance of safety, and by confidence in the efficacy of preventative measures." Although this definition is a bit more technical, I like the fact that it illustrates a food safety culture is made up of both individual and group thoughts, attitudes, and behaviors. It illustrates that food safety is independent. Each employee or person within an organization has a personal responsibility for preparing or serving safe food. It also illustrates that food safety is interdependent. All employees within the whole of the organization or company have a shared responsibility to ensure food safety. And the sum of food safety efforts within an organization is critically dependent on and greater than its parts.

But my all time favorite definition, because of its simplicity, is "Culture is the way we do things around here." Simply put, a food safety culture is how an organization or group does food safety.

Why Is Culture Important?

I want you to pause for a moment and take off your "food safety" hat. Think about a major catastrophic safety accident that you've read about in the newspaper or heard about on the news (Fig. 2.2). Do you recall what the underlying root cause was? Was it reported that the accident was due to faulty design? Was it attributed to operator error? Do you recall if improper training was implicated as the cause?

In major or catastrophic safety accidents of our day, it is not uncommon for the immediate cause to be identified, for example, as faulty design,

> In major safety accident investigations, an underlying root cause is (select one)?
>
> 1. Faulty design
> 2. Operator error
> 3. Improper training
> 4. Organizational culture

Fig. 2.2 Accident investigation root causes

operator error, or improper training. However, if you take a closer look at investigations of major accidents such as Three Mile Island, Chernobyl, and the Shuttle Disaster, an underlying cause – the organization's culture – is often cited as the foundational issue that goes deeper than the immediate or apparent reason. As an important illustration of this point, on February 1, 2003, the United States of America suffered the tragic loss of the Space Shuttle Columbia and its seven-member crew. The physical cause of the accident was determined to be a breach in the Thermal Protection System on the leading edge of the left wing of the shuttle. The damage occurred when a piece of insulating foam separated from the external tank shortly after launch striking the left wing. Although the accident investigation report was exhaustive and detailed, there was one statement in particular in the report that stood out to me. The Columbia Accident Investigation Board (2003) concluded, "In our view, the NASA organizational culture had as much to do with this accident as the foam." This quote serves as a powerful and sobering reminder of the importance of culture.

There is no question that an organization's culture influences how it does safety. The organization's culture will influence how individuals within the group think about safety, their attitudes toward safety, their willingness to openly discuss safety concerns and share differing opinions, and, in general, the emphasis that they place on safety. So is this point also applicable in the field of food safety? Of course it is. However, it's interesting to note that it's uncommon to see reports of foodborne outbreak investigations or other significant food safety events where the organization's culture is even mentioned. I suggest that in some of the major food safety incidents of our day, the organization's culture has also played a key role.

Who Creates Culture?

In an organization or social group, food safety is a shared responsibility. There is no question about it. But when it comes to creating, strengthening, or sustaining a culture within an organization, there is one group of individuals who really own it – they're the leaders.

I came across a quote by Edgar Schein (1992), author on organizational culture, which states this point quite well. He said, "Organizational cultures are created by leaders, and one of the most decisive functions of leadership may well be the creation, the management, and – if and when necessary – the destruction of culture."

Although this quote may strike you as being a bit strong, it's true. The strength of an organization's food safety culture is a direct reflection of how important food safety is to its leadership. A food safety culture starts at the top and flows downward. It is not created from the bottom up. If an organization's food safety culture is less than acceptable, it's the leaders who are ultimately responsible and who own it.

Now, don't think for a minute that I'm implying that a mid-level food safety manager or quality assurance professional within an organization has no role in creating or managing a food safety culture. I'm not suggesting this at all. I've seen this all too often where an ineffective mid-level food safety professional blames senior management on the lack of effectiveness of their food safety efforts. To effectively influence upward, mid-level professionals need to recognize that their goal is to help senior leadership create a food safety culture, not to simply support the food safety programs that they're managing. To do this, they need to thoroughly understand the elements of organizational culture and the dimensions of human behavior. They also need to have effective relationship, communication, and influence skills. Mid level managers are also considered leaders too. And they have a responsibility to effectively advise senior leadership and influence upwards. They also own the culture.

How Is Culture Created?

Having a strong food safety culture is a choice. Ideally, the leaders of an organization will proactively choose to have a strong food safety culture because it's the right thing to do. Safety is a firm value of the organization. Notice that I said "it's a value and not a priority." Priorities can change; values should not (Geller, 2005). The organization chooses to have a strong food safety culture, because it values the safety of its customers and employees. The leaders of the organization have vision and foresight, knowing that having a strong food safety culture is important and that it directly and indirectly benefits the business.

Although less desirable, for other organizations or groups, establishing a strong food safety culture might be driven out of necessity. Their focus on improving their food safety culture is reactionary. It's driven by a significant or major event. They've experienced a food borne illness outbreak, high profile media expose, or an important regulatory issue. They're reacting to pressure.

Regardless of whether it's based on a proactive vision or a reactive event, creating a strong food safety culture does not happen by chance. Simply reading a book on it does not create it, nor will attending a seminar on the topic. And if your organization's food safety culture is already well established and it's less than acceptable, it will not be easy to change. Depending on the circumstances, changing the ingrained thoughts, beliefs and behaviors of a group can be difficult and take several years. Creating or strengthening a food safety culture will require the intentional commitment and hard work by leaders at all levels of the organization starting at the top. But the good news is that it can be done.

The Foundation

Like building a house, a food safety culture built on a solid foundation will be much stronger. And the foundation of an organization is its values. To build an effective food safety culture, an organization or social group should clearly define safety as a foundational value. As mentioned earlier, values are different than priorities (Geller, 2005). Priorities can change depending on circumstances. Values should not. Values are deep seeded principles or beliefs that guide how an organization makes decisions and conducts its business. In many organizations with strong safety cultures, past or present leaders have articulated how much they value safety by crafting a set of guiding safety principles or safety beliefs. They have documented their commitment to safety. But before you jump to a conclusion and think that this sounds like a hokey gimmick or feel-good exercise, think again. Documenting commitments in writing is important. Cialdini (1993) in his classic book, *Influence, The Psychology of Persuasion*, shows that there is scientific evidence that a written commitment is much effective than a verbal one. According to Cialdini (1993), people want to live up to what they've written. By documenting a set of guiding food safety principles or food safety beliefs, the leaders of an organization are increasing the pressure for the actions of the organization or employees to be consistent with its beliefs. They are also making sure that the organization's values or beliefs are clear to all and that they can be shared with others. When creating a food safety culture, this is a good place to start. Call the leaders of the organization together and have them – not you – articulate and craft a set of food safety beliefs or principles.

Core Elements

Although no two great food safety cultures will be identical, they are likely to have many similar attributes. According to a research report by Whiting and Bennett (2003), titled *Driving Towards "0", Best Practices in Corporate Safety and Health, How Leading Companies Develop Safety Cultures*, the safety cultures of 65 leading U.S. Companies had similar core elements. Although the report focused on occupational safety and health issues, let's review some of the elements they identified and how they relate to a food safety culture.

Leadership at the Top

As mentioned earlier in this chapter, a food safety culture starts at the top and flows downward. It does not flow from the bottom up. It is a leadership function to create a food safety vision, set expectations, and inspire others to follow. It's interesting to note that in the field of food safety, we often talk about food safety management. We rarely talk about food safety leadership. But management and leadership are different. According to Maxwell (1998), "the main difference between the two is that leadership is about influencing people to follow, while management focuses on maintaining systems and processes." Leading companies with strong safety cultures not only have strong food safety management systems in place, they also have strong leaders committed to food safety who are able to influence others and lead the way to safer performance.

Confidence in the Part of All Employees

Employees at all levels must be certain that the organization values food safety comparably with its other values. The only way to gain employee confidence is for the leaders of an organization to walk the talk. If the organization claims that the safety of its customers and employees is a company value, rest assured that employees will be watching to make sure that the organization's actions are consistent with the talk. If they perceive any inconsistencies or compromises concerning the organization's commitment to food safety, they will lose trust. And without trust, an organization or leader is no longer credible and unlikely to be followed. Companies with strong safety cultures have earned the confidence of their employees through their actions, not words.

Clear Management Visibility and Leadership

Even if you have strong vision and leadership at the top, without buy-in and support by mid-level management, you cannot have a great food safety culture. Managers at all levels of the organization need to visibly demonstrate their commitment to food safety by the little things they say and do. Every single day, managers at all levels will influence front-line employees whether they realize it or not. If managers have a negative attitude about following proper food safety and sanitation procedures, it will be evident to others by what they say and do. For example, if the manager of a foodservice establishment doesn't wash his hands before beginning work, how can he expect the employees to do so? Instead, if the manager demonstrates a positive attitude toward food safety through his words and action, the employees will more likely do the same. In companies with strong safety cultures, a proper attitude toward food safety is more caught than taught.

Accountability at All Levels

An organization needs to make sure that employees understand the food safety performance expectations of their job and that at all levels they are held accountable for them. The word accountability generally implies that there are checks and balances being measured to make sure certain desired outcomes are being achieved. And in organizations with strong food safety cultures, this is certainly true. For example, an organization might conduct daily HACCP checks and measurements, observe employee behaviors related to food safety, and provide feedback and coaching (both positive and negative) based on the results. But in organizations with enlightened safety cultures, they've figured out a way to transcend or go beyond accountability. They've figured out a way to get employees to do the right things, not because they're being held accountable to them, but because the employees believe in and are committed to food safety. It has been said that character is what you do when you're alone and no one is watching. In organizations with enlightened food safety cultures, employees do the right thing not because the manager or customer is watching, but because they know it's right and they care.

Sharing of Knowledge and Information

The sharing of information and knowledge is like glue that holds a social group together. And organizations with strong safety cultures know this. They take the sharing of information beyond simple food safety training. They share information often and communicate regularly with their employees about food safety using a variety of messages and mediums. They realize that what we see, what we hear, and what we read, if done effectively, can have a tremendous influence on us. If it didn't, advertisers wouldn't spend the millions of dollars they do each year trying to reach consumers. Like in commercial marketing, organizations with strong food safety cultures share information not just to impart knowledge, but to persuade their employees to action.

Best Practices

In addition to the core elements reviewed above, Whiting and Bennett (2003) also identified over 20 best practices among organizations with strong safety cultures as illustrated in Fig. 2.3. Again, although these best practices were related to occupational health and safety issues, many are also applicable to food safety. Best practices ranged from operational integration of safety to managers emphasizing safety as a company value to recognition of superior safety performance.

Practices and Program
- Operational Integration
- Motivational Program
- Behavioral Observation & Feedback
- Safety Committees
- Case Management
- Safety Survey

Managers Required to Show Visibility
- Emphasize as a Company Value
- Discuss Safety at Employee Meetings
- Participate in Safety Committees
- Do Frequent "Walk Arounds"
- Ensure Adequate Resources
- Ensure Employee Training
- Create Trusting Relationships
- Suspend Unsafe Activities

Front Line Supervisor Responsibilities
- Encourage Safe/Discourage Unsafe Behaviors
- Conduct hazard analysis
- Train Employees
- Conduct Documented Safety Inspections
- Investigate Incidents & Near Misses

Employee Involvement
- Safety Performance Objectives
- Recognition of Superior Safety Performance
- Progressive Discipline for Unsafe Practices

Fig. 2.3 Safety culture best practices

Although identifying best practices can be useful, one major drawback to creating such a list is that it doesn't really demonstrate how these activities are linked together or interrelated. In fact, this same mistake is often made by food safety professionals who benchmark with other organizations to identify a list of food safety best practices for potential implementation within their own company or place of employment. The problem with this type of approach is that it oversimplifies food safety efforts. It approaches food safety like a cafeteria with a list of potential menu options without understanding how the various best practices might be linked together or how they might influence each other. It misses or oversimplifies where these best practices or efforts fit into the bigger picture – the system.

To effectively create or sustain a food safety culture, it is critical to have a systems thinking mindset. You must realize the interdependency of each of the various efforts your organization chooses to put into practice and how the totality of those efforts might influence people's thoughts and behaviors. In order to create a food safety culture, you need to have *a systems-based approach to food safety*. This is the topic of the next chapter.

Key Points

- The goal of the food safety professional should be to create a food safety culture – not a food safety program.

- Culture is patterned ways of thought and behaviors that characterize a social group which can be learned through socialization processes and persist through time.
- An organization's culture will influence how individuals within the group think about food safety, their attitudes toward food safety, their willingness to openly discuss concerns and share differing opinions, and, in general, the emphasis that they place on food safety.
- When it comes to creating, strengthening, or sustaining a food safety culture within an organization, there is one group of individuals who really own it – they're the leaders.
- Having a strong food safety culture is a choice. The leaders of an organization should proactively choose to have a strong food safety culture because it's the right thing to do, as opposed to reacting to a significant issue or outbreak.
- Creating or strengthening a food safety culture will require the intentional commitment and hard work by leaders at all levels of the organization, starting at the top.
- Although no two great food safety cultures will be identical, they are likely to have many similar attributes.
- Identifying food safety best practices can be useful, but one major drawback to creating such a list is that it doesn't really demonstrate how these activities are linked together or interrelated. It misses the big picture – the system.
- To create a food safety culture, you need to have *a systems-based approach to food safety*.

Chapter 3
A Systems-Based Approach to Food Safety

> *A system is an entity, which maintains its existence through the mutual interaction of its parts.*
> Ludwig von Bertalanffy, Austrian Biologist (1901–1972)

Today's professional in pursuit of food safety excellence will find a host of articles, books, and conferences describing a wide range of activities, which they can consider implementing within their organization or place of employment. If you've ever attended a food safety seminar or conference, you'll know what I mean. Some of the activities discussed can range from specific training programs for line-level employees to the types of inspections conducted by food safety professionals to the adoption of electronic information technology systems. While all of these topics are important, one major drawback to approaching food safety in this manner is that it doesn't demonstrate how the many activities an organization may choose to implement are linked together or interrelated. It doesn't demonstrate how they might influence each other. And the biggest drawback of all is that it doesn't adequately consider how the totality of those efforts might influence people's thoughts and behaviors. It doesn't treat the totality of food safety efforts as a *system*. It misses the big picture.

While I realize that in the field of food safety today the term *food safety management system* is commonly used, it is not generally used in the context referred to in this textbook. The term food safety management system usually refers to a system that includes having prerequisite programs in place, good manufacturing practices (GMPs), a Hazard Analysis of Critical Control Point plan, a recall procedure, and so on. It's a very process focused system. Don't get me wrong, I'm all for well-defined processes and standards. They're critical. But having well-defined processes and standards isn't enough. The system referred to in this book is a different sort of system. It's not only process focused, but it's also people focused. It's a total systems approach based on the scientific knowledge of human behavior, organizational culture, and food safety. I'll refer to it as a *behavior-based food safety management system*.

Remember, at the end of the day, to improve the food safety performance of an organization, you have to change people's behaviors. You can have the best-documented food safety processes and standards in the world, but if they are not consistently put into practice by people, they're useless. Accordingly, our system has to address both the science of food safety and the dimensions of organizational culture and human behavior.

What Is a System?

In order to have a systems thinking mindset, we must first understand what a system is. According to Webster's dictionary (1985), *a system is a regularly interacting or interdependent group of items forming a unified whole*. If you think about it, systems are quite common and they're everywhere. They range from simple systems to the more complex systems of life. There are living systems and there are non-living systems. Examples of living systems include a single cell, our central nervous system, a person, an ecosystem, or even an organization. Systems thinkers are generally focused on living systems, such as biological or human social systems. In our case, the unified whole or the system that we're concerned about is the organization's food safety culture – the way an organization does food safety or the patterned ways of thoughts and behaviors about food safety demonstrated by employees in the organization. The food safety culture is a likely part of a larger system, the overall culture of the organization. But for our purposes, we'll stay focused specifically on the food safety culture.

Systems Thinking

As we have acquired scientific knowledge through research and analytical methodologies about the causes of food borne disease, food safety professionals have advanced food safety through the implementation of specific risk management strategies. At times, specific food safety concerns and strategies have been studied and tackled in isolation, as individual components, not as a whole or complete system. Although this sort of linear cause-and-effect thinking in many instances has served us well, it is not fully adequate to address some of the challenges we face, including those related to an organization's food safety culture or an employee's adherence to food safety practices and behaviors. This is because these issues involve multiple components that are interrelated.

A critical characteristic of a system is that it cannot be fully explained or understood by simply studying each of its components in isolation. It must be explained by understanding how each part or component interacts and influences other components. Webster's definition of a system used above, where the *parts of the system interact and are interdependent,* suggests something beyond a simple cause-and-effect relationship. For example, instead of component A simply affecting component B (Fig. 3.1), component B may also affect component A directly or indirectly (Fig. 3.2). A system calls for a more complex understanding of relatedness, such as feedback relationships, to explain the role of the various components in the system as a whole.

Only by acquiring a systems-thinking mindset, can we as food safety professionals adequately develop a *behavior-based food safety management system*.

3 A Systems-Based Approach to Food Safety

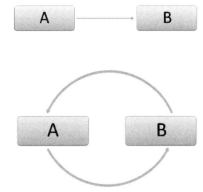

Fig. 3.1 Simple linear cause and effect relationship

Fig. 3.2 Simple system feedback relationship

Behavior Change Theories and Models

Changing behaviors, especially those related to health and safety, can be difficult. Before we proceed with developing a blueprint for creating a total systems-based approach to food safety, we should note that there are numerous theories published specifically on behavior change. Although this book or chapter is not intended to provide an exhaustive review of behavioral change theories, as a food safety professional, you should be aware of them. Accordingly, a brief summary of some of the more prominent theories recognized by public health professionals is listed below.

Behavioral Theory

Behavioral theory is largely based on B.F. Skinner's (1953) work on operant conditioning. According to this theory, changes in behavior are a response to stimuli in the environment. The theory is based on the pairing of the desired response or behavior with a reinforcer. Repeated pairing of the desired behavior with a positive or negative reinforcer can either increase or decrease the behavior. For example, an employee who gives a customer outstanding service may get a recognition card (with value) from the supervisor. The card is intended as positive reinforcement to strengthen the likelihood that the behavior will occur again. In contrast, an employee who breaks a company policy may get a written reprimand intended to stop the undesired behavior.

Social Cognitive Theory

According to cognitive theories, humans are more complex than a series of responses to external stimuli. Social cognitive theory emphasizes that behaviors are influenced by the environment and personal factors (Baranowski, Perry, &

Parcel, 2002). A person's behavior will be influenced by their beliefs, attitudes, and perceptions. Central concepts in the social cognitive theory are those of skills and self-efficacy. If a person perceives an incentive related to a specific behavior, they must believe they are capable of performing it (self-efficacy). Success at performing the behavior enhances the probability that the behavior will be performed again.

Health Belief Model

The Health Belief Model is one that is commonly used by public health professionals when dealing with health-related behaviors. It is based on four key concepts (Janz, Champion, & Stretcher, 2002). The first is an individual's perception of their susceptibility or risk of contracting an illness or disease. For example, if based on family history, a person believes they are at increased risk for cancer; they may be more likely to listen to health advice. The second key concept is the person's perception of how severe the illness or condition could be. Illnesses and conditions that are not very severe are less likely to get someone's attention. The third concept is a person's perception of the benefits of taking some form of preventive action. If a person doubts the effectiveness of a remedy or recommended solution, they are unlikely to follow it. And lastly, the fourth key concept relates to a person's perceived barrier to taking action. Barriers can be varied and they include language, cultural, financial, and others. For example, if a person perceives that eating healthy costs more, they may be less likely to change to their dietary purchasing habits.

Theory of Reasoned Action

The primary focus of the Theory of Reasoned Action is on attitudes, beliefs, and intentions. According to this theory, a person's intention to perform a specific behavior is motivated primarily by their intention (Montano & Kasprzyk, 2002). A person's intentions, their health beliefs, are influenced by two key factors. One, their level of intention is greater if they have a positive attitude about the behavior. Second, their level of intention is greater if they are motivated to comply with a social norm.

Transtheoretical Model

The Transtheoretical Model explains behavior change as a series of six stages a person goes through related to their readiness to change. The stages are pre-contemplation, contemplation, preparation, action, maintenance, and termination (Prochaska & DiClemente, 1986). Using this theory, specific interventions to influence behavior change should match the stage the person is in or their state of readiness to change.

Social Marketing

Although Social Marketing is not a behavioral theory it is a set of procedures that can be used to promote change related to health behaviors. As defined by Andreasen (1995), "social marketing is the application of commercial marketing technologies to the analysis, planning, execution, and evaluation of programs designed to influence the voluntary behavior of target audiences in order to improve their personal welfare and that of society."

Environmental or Physical Factors

An important element of behavioral change, which is often missing in behavior change theories and models, is the importance of environmental or physical factors, such as facility design, equipment selection, and work tools, on a person's willingness to engage in certain behaviors. In other words, these environmental or physical factors are part of the overall system and they influence a person's behaviors and actions. As illustrated in Fig. 3.3, Geller (2005) indicates that physical factors are one of three principle components of a safety system. As yet another example of the importance of this principle, in a model published by the Centers for Disease Control and Prevention, National Center for Environmental Health, Environmental Health Services (Fig. 3.4), physical factors are one of four major components of an overall food safety system.

Clearly, when it comes to food safety management, having the fundamental physical components of the system in place is critical. Facilities should be designed with food safety and sanitation in mind and they must comply with all relevant regulatory standards. The right equipment must be selected for the

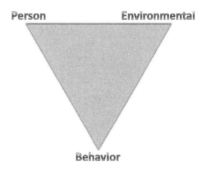

Fig. 3.3 Environment, behavior, and personal factors affecting safety (Geller)

Fig. 3.4 Food safety system (Centers for Disease Control and Prevention, National Center for Environmental Health, Environmental Health Services)

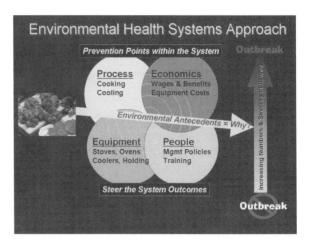

right job. And employees must be provided with the proper tools necessary to do their work. To illustrate this point, let's highlight just a few critical physical components as required by the (2001) Food and Drug Administration Food Code. In retail food establishments, floors, floor coverings, walls, wall coverings, and ceilings shall be designed, constructed, and installed so they are smooth and easily cleanable. Outer openings of a food establishment shall be protected against the entry of insects and rodents by filling or closing holes and other gaps along floors, walls, and ceilings; closed, tight-fitting windows; and solid, self-closing, tight-fitting doors. Equipment and utensils shall be designed and constructed to be durable and to retain their characteristic qualities under normal use conditions. And a hand washing facility shall be located to allow convenient use by employees in food preparation, food dispensing, and ware washing areas; and in, or immediately adjacent to, toilet rooms. Since the physical requirements in the Food Code are too numerous to list here, suffice it to say that having the right physical components in place is foundational to an effective food safety management system.

Not unexpectedly, often times, environmental or physical factors are directly or indirectly linked to behavior. As a simple example, let's consider the behavior of hand washing. If employees are expected to wash their hands before starting work and in between certain tasks, even if employees have been trained on the importance of hand washing, having a hand sink that is conveniently located will increase the chances that the employees will actually do so. Imagine a scenario where the employees are extremely busy and barely have enough time to keep up with work orders. Do you think they will consistently take the time to go wash their hands if they have to leave the work area, travel a long distance, and get behind in their work?

But facility design, equipment selection, and work tools are not always sufficient to explain behavior. To make this point, let's revisit the behavior of hand washing. What do you think motivates a person to wash their hands after using the restroom? Is it simply the fact that they have a hand sink that is conveniently located, functional, and properly designed? How many times have you been in a public restroom that had a touch-free, functional hand sink, which was conveniently located; yet you saw someone use the restroom and leave it without washing his or her hands? I'm sure you've experienced this. It's quite common. In fact, according to a study published by the American Society of Microbiology (2005), 91% of American adults said they always wash their hands after using public restrooms, but when observed in such settings, only 83% actually did so. In many cases, the unsafe or undesired behavior – in this case a person choosing to not wash their hands after using the restroom – is not due to the facility being improperly designed or because hand sinks are not conveniently located. The reason for the unsafe behavior is due to other factors – not physical ones. A person's willingness to use the hand sink, often times goes beyond facility design or having the right tools. It's more complex than that. Often times, to drive, shape, and achieve the desired behavior; we need to consider other elements of the system – not just the physical ones.

A Behavior-Based Systems Continuous Improvement Model

For the remainder of this book, let's assume that having well-designed facilities, proper equipment, and the right work tools, is foundational to effective food safety management. We won't spend a lot of time on this, since there are numerous contributions to this subject in the scientific literature as well as in regulatory, equipment, and design standards. For the remainder of this book, I will focus on select, non-physical components of the system responsible for creating a food safety culture.

They say a picture is worth a thousand words. Well, if that's the case, then a model is worth ten thousand. The illustration in Fig. 3.5 depicts a continuous

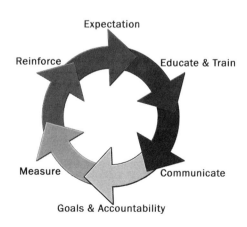

Fig. 3.5 Behavior-based food safety management system continuous improvement model

improvement model for select, non-physical concepts and activities responsible for creating a *behavior-based food safety management system*. Although the model is not intended to be all-inclusive, it should serve as a useful framework of some of the more critical components, which should be considered when attempting to create or strengthen a food safety culture.

Key Points

- In the field of food safety today the term *food safety management system* is commonly used, but it is not used in the context referred to in this textbook. The term food safety management system usually is very process focused.
- A *behavior-based food safety management system* is process focused, but it's also people focused. It's a total systems approach based on the scientific knowledge of human behavior, organizational culture, and food safety.
- A system is a regularly interacting or interdependent group of items forming a unified whole.
- A system cannot be explained using simple linear cause-and-effect thinking. It requires a more complex understanding of relatedness, such as feedback relationships, to explain the role of the various components in the system as a whole.
- A systems thinking mindset is required to adequately develop a *behavior-based food safety management system*.
- Changing behaviors, especially those related to health and safety can be difficult. Food safety professionals should be familiar some of the more prominent behavioral change theories and models including Behavioral Theory, Social Cognitive Theory, Health Belief Model, Theory of Reasoned Action, Transtheoretical Model, and Social Marketing.
- An important element of behavioral change, which is often missing in behavior change theories and models, is the importance of environmental or physical factors, such as facility design, equipment selection, and work tools, on a person's willingness to engage in certain behaviors.
- A *behavior-based food safety management system* can be created using continuous improvement model.

Chapter 4
Creating Food Safety Performance Expectations

> *The quality of expectations determines the quality of our actions.*
>
> A. Godin, French Writer (1880–1938)

When it comes to desired food safety performance by employees, many professionals think that the first step in achieving conformance is to make sure all employees receive proper food safety training. Others think that the key to conformance is to regularly inspect retail food establishments for certain behaviors, outcomes, or conditions. In fact, training and inspections are two of the most commonly used tools by food safety professionals when attempting to achieve a desired performance objective. But training and inspections are not the first steps in this process, nor are they the only steps in this process – and they are certainly not enough. Achieving excellence in food safety performance actually starts earlier than this. It begins with creating food safety performance expectations that are clear, achievable, and understood by all. In other words, if an organization wants to achieve excellence in the area of food safety, employees at all levels need to know what is expected of them and what exactly they must do to achieve it. This is the first step in creating a behavior-based food safety management system.

Getting Employees to Do What They Are Supposed to Do

Getting employees to do what you want them to do is not easy. And some believe it's getting even harder. Many consultants cite that the work force is changing. They say that, in general, there has been a loss of respect for authority figures, which include managers and supervisors at work. Others say that the work ethic in this country is declining. They say employees just don't care about work or doing a good job like they used to. But are there other critical reasons why employees don't perform as desired by employers? As unbelievable as this may sound, according to Fournies (1999), the most common reason managers give as to why people at work don't do what they are supposed to do is, "they don't know what they are supposed to do." Think about this. One of the main reasons employees don't perform as desired is because they don't know what is expected of them. Employees need to have clear and achievable food safety performance expectations that define what it is that they must do and how they are to fulfill such tasks. Of interest, many managers and leaders will spend time on clearly defining performance expectations with employees, but only after there appears to be a performance problem. Defining expectations once performance problems arise is too late – especially when it comes to food safety. Performance expectations need to be defined and shared with employees in advance of them performing assigned duties and tasks, so that they are set up for success and do them safely.

In addition to making sure expectations are clear and achievable, they should also be of high quality. As a manager, you'll get what you expect. If your expectations are unclear, employees won't know what you want them to do. If they're clear, but low, you'll get mediocre results. In contrast, if your expectations are clear, high, and uncompromising, you'll achieve more. According to the late Sam Walton, founder of Wal-Mart Stores, Inc., "high expectations are the key to everything." As an astute businessman filled with wisdom and common sense, Sam knew that the quality of his expectations would determine the quality of the actions of those around him. And with clear and high expectations, he was able to create what some considered unimaginable – the world's largest retail chain with over one million associates.

Expect More than Efficiency

In today's fast-paced business world, many retail food organizations are focused on doing things more efficiently. If there is one single word or thought that I would choose to describe today's retail food world, it's the word *more*. There are more demands by customers. There are more products or options to choose from. Consumers are eating more and more meals outside the home (in retail food establishments). There are more foodborne concerns, more regulations, and often times all of this translates into *more* work to do by employees in retail food establishments. Accordingly, many organizations are focused on doing things more efficiently. But in addition to the focus on doing more (or doing things more efficiently), we should be equally focused on doing things right. Of the many fields or disciplines where expectations should be clear, high, and uncompromising (so that things are done right), the field of retail food safety is certainly one of them. Think about it, when it comes to food safety, almost right or pretty good may not be good enough. Imagine a situation where employees don't know that they are expected to thoroughly cook hamburger patties and how they are to perform this task. Do you think they will consistently do so? How about a scenario where cooking burgers to "almost" the right temperature, just slightly undercooked, is tolerated as good enough. If the burgers are contaminated with *E. coli* 0157:H7, it can result in tragic results. When it comes to food safety, establishing well-defined performance expectations is critical. Without them, you won't consistently get the right actions, outcomes, or results.

Expect a Proper Food Safety Attitude

When creating food safety expectations, one of the first places to start is to expect employees to have a proper food safety attitude, which aligns with the organization's beliefs and values. Now, I understand that you can't force people to have the right food safety attitude, but you certainly can expect it and model it. For example, is it the general attitude of those in the organization that all foodborne illnesses are preventable or is it believed that some foodborne illnesses are unavoidable? Establishing an expectation that foodborne illnesses are preventable clearly communicates to each employee in the organization that they are expected to do their part in making safe food and keeping it safe.

Do team members in the organization think that a certain number of critical violations per inspection is acceptable or have they adopted the organization's zero-tolerance philosophy believing that one critical violation is one critical violation too many. I realize we live in an imperfect world and that there is no such thing as perfection, but organizations and individuals who are always striving to get better are the ones that usually do. In general, an organization will get more of what it tolerates. If an organization tolerates two or three critical violations per inspection, they'll get stores that are operated at a level of food safety and sanitation performance where two or three critical violations per inspection is the norm. If an organization operates under a zero-tolerance philosophy toward critical violations, critical violations will be less common and the team will probably be striving to get better.

Expect employees to have a right attitude about food safety, because an employee with a right attitude will be much more likely to take right actions. Also, every single day, each employee will influence those around him or her, whether we realize it or not. If they have a negative attitude about following proper food safety and sanitation procedures, trust me – it will be evident to others by what they say and do. Instead, if they demonstrate a positive attitude toward food safety, food safety performance will increase exponentially because of their positive influence on others around them.

Be Specific – Not Generic

When it comes to food safety performance, a common mistake retail food organizations often make is to be vague or unclear on what they expect their employees to do. Food safety performance expectations should be clear and specific – not generic. Forget the cute and catchy slogans to describe what you want your employees to do. Although slogans such as "food safety, it's in your hands" or "think safety" may sound catchy, they're not very effective. What do they mean? It doesn't tell an employee what it is that they must do to keep food safe. Ideally, food safety performance expectations should be objective, observable, and related to specific tasks and behaviors.

Fig. 4.1 FDA food code table of contents (2001)

Chapter 1	Purpose and Definitions
Chapter 2	Management and Personnel
Chapter 3	Food
Chapter 4	Equipment, Utensils, and Linens
Chapter 5	Water, Plumbing, and Waste
Chapter 6	Physical Facilities
Chapter 7	Poisonous or Toxic Materials
Chapter 8	Compliance and Enforcement

Over the years, I've been able to talk to employees of retail food establishments all over the country and world. And when I talk to them about food safety, I find many who are genuinely interested in trying to do the right thing. But they're looking for more than simply being admonished with catchy slogans to think about food safety. They're looking for specifics on what it is that they must do to keep foods safe. Forget the cute phrases or fancy slogans unless you're going to back them up with specifics. Tell your employees in clear and user-friendly language exactly what they need to do to prepare and serve safe food.

Start with the Food Code

When it comes to creating food safety performance expectations, in the United States, the Food and Drug Administration Food Code (2001) is a good starting point. The stated purpose of the Code is *to safeguard public health and provide to consumers food that is safe, unadulterated, and honestly presented*. The Food Code is the cumulative and collaborative work of many individuals, agencies, and organizations. For businesses, it should be viewed as more than just a regulatory document. It should be viewed as a useful, science-based guide for establishing food safety performance expectations for the organization and its employees. Although the Food Code addresses a broad range of issues as shown in Fig. 4.1, a majority of the behavior-based food safety performance expectations that should be known by and expected of retail food employees can be found in Chapters 2 and 3. These chapters deal with issues ranging from employee health to personal hygiene (including hands as vehicles of food borne disease) to time and temperature requirements for controlling food borne pathogens.

Develop Risk-Based Expectations

Like in many areas of life, when creating food safety performance expectations, you need to establish priorities. In any specific retail food role, there can be numerous duties that an employee will be expected to do. Of those, the tasks, practices, and behaviors that have been scientifically associated with foodborne disease should be the ones where the expectations of how to do them properly are clearly defined. In other words, create food safety performance expectations that are risk-based.

Good foodborne diseases surveillance data and the associated contributing factors of food borne disease are often regarded as important information that is needed by regulatory agencies to better establish regulatory priorities, assist with the allocation of resources, and provide the basis for enactment of new laws and regulations (Guzewich, Bryan, & Todd, 1997). But this same information is also extremely valuable to the industry. In fact, it provides the basis on which industry can rationally establish food safety risk management strategies and priorities – including performance expectations.

As shown in Fig. 4.2, epidemiological outbreak data reported by the Centers for Disease Control and Prevention (Olsen et al., 2000) summarize five major risk factors most commonly contributing to foodborne disease in retail food establishments. These risk factors are linked to many preparation practices and tasks performed by employees. They are also linked to specific employee behaviors. Therefore, it is critical that expectations related to these risk factors be clearly defined and communicated. Since the risk factors are categorized in fairly broad terms, such as *poor personal hygiene* or *inadequate holding temperatures*, there will be multiple tasks and behaviors related to each risk factor.

When creating food safety performance expectations, it is always better to specify them for specific tasks and behaviors related to the foodborne risk factor than for the generic foodborne risk factor itself. For example as shown in Fig. 4.3, rather than stating *employees must follow good personal hygiene*, tell them exactly what that means. Specifically, employees should know that if they're experiencing (or have recently experienced) gastrointestinal symptoms such as nausea, vomiting, fever, or diarrhea, they must not work with food, drinks,

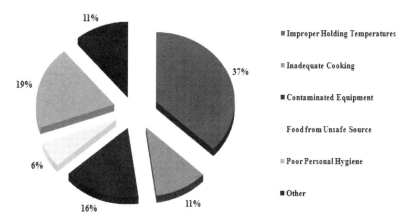

Fig. 4.2 Number of foodborne outbreaks in the United States by contributing factor (CDC, 1993–1997) (*See* Color Insert)

Foodborne Risk Factor (Generic)	Expected Behaviors (Specific)
Poor Personal Hygiene	Do not work with food if ill with gastrointestinal symptoms such as nausea, vomiting, fever, or diarrhea
	Do not contact ready-to-eat foods with bare hands. Instead, use single service gloves, deli tissue, or other suitable utensil.
	Wash your hands thoroughly with soap and warm water in a designated hand sink before starting your shift or returning from a break; after using the restroom; before and after changing single use gloves; after coughing, sneezing, or using a handkerchief; and before working with food, beverages, or utensils.

Fig. 4.3 Specific behaviors related to risk factors

equipment, or utensils. They should know that they must not contact ready-to-eat foods with their bare hands. Instead, for the specific task or food in question, they should know whether they are to use single service gloves, deli tissue, or other suitable utensil. They should know when and how to wash their hands. It should be a clear expectation that they cannot eat, drink, chew gum, or smoke in food preparation, storage, and warewashing areas. And so on and so on.

As another illustration, instead of telling employees to *keep foods at proper temperatures*, tell them exactly what this means. For example, check temperatures of perishable foods upon receipt and document the temperature on the packing slip. File the packing slip for a minimum of 30 days. Reject foods that are not received at 41° F or below. Refrigerate food promptly upon receiving. Keep cold foods cold at 41° F or below and keep hot foods hot at 140° F or higher. You should specify how they are to take food temperatures, how often, where to document it, and what to do if the temperatures do not meet a defined standard. And so on and so on.

Beyond Regulatory Compliance

Although regulatory standards are getting tougher, they are generally considered a minimum standard. When developing the food safety performance expectations for an organization, think about more than regulatory standards (as defined in the Food Code) and the Centers for Disease Control and Prevention's foodborne risk factors. Think about other issues related to food safety.

As an illustration of this point, let's consider food allergies. Food allergies are increasing and, in the United States are reported to account for an estimated 30,000 emergency room visits and up to 200 deaths each year. The current consensus among scientists is that about 12 million Americans suffer from a food allergy. With this many Americans suffering from food allergies, as you can imagine, many of them are eating out at retail food establishments. In fact, several published studies have shown that food allergic reactions occur in restaurants, some leading to death. Although food allergies are often times not addressed in regulatory standards, employees of retail food establishments should have expectations clearly defined for them concerning food allergies. For example, front-line employees and waiters or waitresses should know that if they get questions related to food allergies, they should stop, take them very seriously, and get the chef or person in charge to address them. Managers and chefs in the organization should know the foods identified as major allergens, how to reduce the likelihood of cross contact between allergy-free and allergy-containing food, and so on.

As yet another expectation that is rarely found in regulatory standards, let's consider the topic of food defense, sometimes also referred to as food security. Do employees in the organization know what is expected of them regarding food products returned by a customer, regardless of whether or not it is in a sealed or unopened package? Do they clearly understand what they are expected to do if they detect an unfamiliar or unauthorized person in a kitchen or food warehouse area?

Clearly, when creating food safety performance expectations for an organization, you must think beyond mere regulatory compliance. Think about all the things that employees should know related to risk and food – and clearly define what you want them to do.

Write Them All Down

Food safety performance expectations should be documented, so that they are clear and communicated in a consistent manner. At a minimum, food safety performance expectations should be captured in one central document. Better yet, they can also be integrated with other expectations such as in operational manuals or procedures.

As previously stated, although the Food Code and foodborne disease risk factors can serve as useful, science-based guides for establishing food safety performance expectations, they are not written in simple, user-friendly terms that employees are likely to understand. In fact, the Food Code is a 600 plus pages long document, fairly technical, and unlikely to be easily understood by employees. Accordingly, you'll have to write down the food safety performance expectations for your organization in a manner, which will be easily understood by your employees.

There are four guiding principles that should be followed when writing food safety performance expectations as listed in Fig. 4.4. One, food safety performance expectations should be *simple*. To make things simple, often times, this

> Food safety performance expectations should be **simple**.
>
> Food safety performance expectations should be **clear**.
>
> Food safety performance expectations should be **risk-based.**
>
> Food safety performance expectations should be **relevant.**

Fig. 4.4 Food safety performance expectations guiding principles

requires a lot of effort. Complicated expectations or tasks are less likely to be understood or performed correctly. Every effort should be made to engineer or set up work, so that it's simple and uncomplicated. This will increase the chances that the expectation is understood and that it will be performed correctly. Two, food safety performance expectations should be *clear*. If expectations are clear, employees will be much more likely to understand what is expected of them and how to achieve it. Three, food safety performance expectations should be *risk-based*. If expectations are risk-based (and they're followed), the likelihood of food borne disease will be decreased. And four, food safety performance expectations should be *relevant*. If expectations are relevant, employees will understand why they are being asked to do them and it will increase the chances that they will buy into them and do them well.

Once you've identified and documented all of the food safety performance expectations for your organization, you have to share them with your employees and, for some expectations; you'll need to provide education and training. That's the next step in creating a behavior-based food safety management system.

Key Points

- One of the main reasons employees don't perform as desired is because they don't know what is expected of them.
- The first step in creating a *behavior-based food safety management system* is to make sure that food safety performance expectations are clear, achievable, and understood by all.
- Food safety expectations should not only be clear and achievable, they should also be of high quality. The quality of your expectations will influence the quality of your actions and those around you.
- Expect employees to have a proper attitude about food safety, which aligns with the organization's beliefs and values, because a proper attitude increases the chances of right actions.
- Food safety performance expectations should be clear and specific – not generic. Forget about cute and catchy slogans to describe what you want your employees to do, unless you back them with specifics.

Color Insert

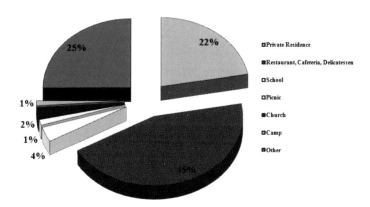

Fig. 1.5 Number of reported foodborne outbreaks in the United States by place (CDC, 1993–1997)

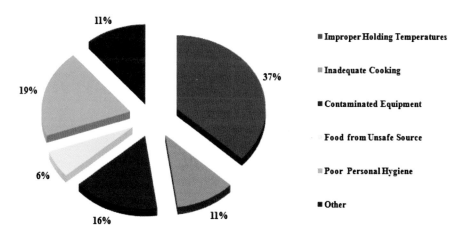

Fig. 1.7 Number of reported foodborne outbreaks in the United States by contributing factor (CDC, 1993–1997)

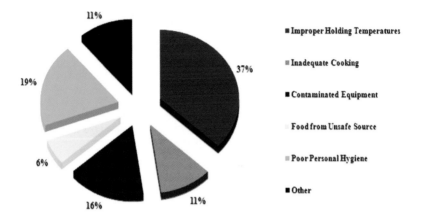

Fig. 4.2 Number of foodborne outbreaks in the United States by contributing factor (CDC, 1993–1997)

- In the United States, the Food and Drug Administration Food Code can be a useful, science-based guide for establishing food safety performance expectations.
- Of the numerous duties that an employee will be expected to do, make sure those tasks, practices, and behaviors that have been scientifically associated with foodborne disease are the ones where the expectations of how to do them properly are clearly defined.
- Ideally, food safety performance expectations should address issues beyond mere regulatory compliance, such as food defense and food allergies.
- To make sure food safety performance expectations are clear and communicated in a consistent manner, they should be documented

Chapter 5
Educating and Training to Influence Behavior

> *I cannot teach anybody anything; I can only make them think.*
> Socrates (470 BC–399 BC)

When it comes to trying to achieve a particular set of desired food safety related behaviors or a certain level of food safety performance, food safety professionals often turn to training as the solution. In fact, training (along with testing and inspections) is one of three of the most commonly used tools in the field of food safety. This point is illustrated by a survey of nationally recognized food safety experts in the United States (Sertkaya, Berlind, Lange, & Zink, 2006). This panel of experts was asked to list the top ten food safety problems in the United States. As shown in Fig. 5.1, of all the potential problems this panel has listed, deficient employee training was listed as number one.

But is food safety training really the number one problem or the silver bullet that it is often implied to be? I think many food safety professionals can relate to a situation where an employee has been properly trained on how to do something, yet fails to do it. Why is that? Well, it's because changing behaviors is really not as simple as just providing training. What we know does not always equal what we do. If it did, many of us would eat less and drive slower. Behavior change can be a difficult and complex process. Now don't get me wrong, I'm not against training. I realize that it is absolutely critical. However, I realize that training must be viewed in its proper context as it relates to behavior change and that it is only one of a series of interactive components of a behavior-based food safety management system.

This chapter is not intended to be a compressive review of training strategies or training principles. There are numerous contributions to the literature on these subjects. One such reference that you might want to review is the Occupational Safety and Health Administration's Training Guideline (OSHA, 1998). Although this guideline is written to address occupational health and safety issues, their training model as outlined in Fig. 5.2 can be used to address food safety concerns too.

Instead, for the remainder of this chapter, we will review several important concepts, which I believe should be considered when evaluating the role of training in a behavior-based food safety management system.

Food Safety Problem	Percentage Vote
Deficient employee training	94%
Contamination of raw material	75%
Poor plant and equipment sanitation	75%
Poor plant design and construction	75%
No preventative maintenance	69%
Difficult to clean equipment	63%
Post process contamination at plant	63%
Contamination during processing	56%
Poor personal hygiene	56%
Incorrect labeling	44%
Contamination by reworked product	31%
Inadequate cooling	31%
Biofilms	25%
Lack of equipment knowledge	25%
Poor pest control	25%
Stagnant water due to dead ends in plumbing	25%
Condensate on pipes and equipment	19%

Fig. 5.1 Ranking of food safety problems by number of votes across all sectors (Sertkaya et al., 2006)

- Determining if Training is Needed
- Identifying Training Needs
- Identifying Goals and Objectives
- Developing Learning Activities
- Conducting the Training
- Evaluating Program Effectiveness
- Improving the Program

Fig. 5.2 Occupational safety and health administration's training model (1998)

Education Versus Training

In the field of food safety, we often talk about food safety training. For example, we talk about food safety training programs, food safety training strategies, and food safety training certifications. However, we rarely talk about food safety education. But training and education are different. In fact, I believe that in our profession today, these terms are often used incorrectly. Much of what is called food safety training today is really food safety education. Remember, the words we use and how we use them are important. So let's take a moment to review the differences between food safety training and food safety education.

I like to describe the differences between food safety training and food safety education like this. Food safety education generally involves the transfer of information related to food safety such as foodborne hazards, regulatory standards, and company policies to a group of individuals or employees. It's generally done by an instructor in a class room setting. For example, an instructor might teach a group of employees about safe food temperatures, potentially hazardous food groups, and specific microbes associated with foodborne disease. More and more today, this practice of educating individuals on food safety is occurring via computers. In fact, it's often referred to as computer-based training. But in reality, whether it's done in a classroom or on a computer, it's education and not training. In general, food safety education involves more of the *why* food safety is important than the *how to do* food safety.

Food safety training is different. It involves more of the *how* than the *why*. It is generally one-on-one, hands-on, specific, and on-the-job. It involves teaching employees the details of tasks or duties assigned to them through demonstration and how they must do them to keep foods safe or make them safe. For example, a supervisor or lead might teach a new employee how to use a chain broiler, with food safety principles in mind, before they let them work at this station alone. After they're taught how to use it, the supervisor might ask the new employee to perform the tasks while he or she watches to make sure they've mastered the technique. This is food safety training. It's very specific to certain tasks, integrated with operational responsibilities, and hands-on.

Now, you may be asking yourself, which one is more important, food safety education or food safety training? They both are. It's important to teach the "why" food safety is important in an attempt to transfer knowledge and influence attitudes. But it's equally important to teach the "how" food safety is performed through specific demonstration of tasks and duties assigned to employees. If you only educate, but don't train, you're asking for trouble.

Why Educate and Train?

Before training and education is identified as the solution to achieve a particular outcome or behavior, a thorough needs-assessment should be performed. There are various reasons why an organization may choose to provide food safety training and education to their employees. Besides the fact that it may be a regulatory requirement, an organization may voluntarily choose to provide food safety education and training to provide employees with the knowledge or skills needed to do their job. They might also want to change employee attitudes. All are important and noteworthy goals. Knowledgeable employees are more likely to do what is expected of them. Employees clearly need to have the right skills needed to do their job and keep foods safe. And having the right attitude about food safety is important, because a right attitude increases the chances of right actions. But simply put, the most important reason we should educate and train is to influence behavior.

Focus on Changing Behavior

We all know that behavior change can be complex. So when designing food safety training and education materials, make sure you design it in a persuasive manner with behavior change in mind. So how can you do this? Well, here are two good tips.

First, make sure you understand that a person's perceived risk of an issue is a very good indicator of their willingness to engage in such a practice or behavior. Accordingly, it is critical that employees understand that when it comes to food safety, there are *real risks with real consequences*. For example, if you're trying to persuade an employee about the importance of hand washing, but they have poor hand washing habits and do not see the negative consequences of such poor practices, they will be hard to reach. When educating and training employees, you should stress the seriousness of not following proper practices and their potential consequences. But you'll have to do this tactfully and in a credible manner. If it comes across as alarmist, it can backfire.

Second, when you are designing food safety training and educational materials, realize that personal testimonials or individual case studies are much more persuasive than group statistics (Slovic, 1991). This is an important point, because I find that many food safety professionals frequently try to persuade others on the importance of food safety through the use of foodborne disease statistics rather than individual stories. Personal testimonies can be very powerful. Often times, the listener can relate to the story and put themselves in the other person's shoes. In contrast, they really can't do this with statistics. To make this point, let me illustrate. Which one do you think is more persuasive in getting your attention on the potential seriousness and importance of food allergies? The food allergy statistics listed in Fig. 5.3 or the personal testimony by a mother who lost her daughter due to an avoidable food allergic reaction (Fig. 5.4)? And when personal testimonies are told via video rather than by the written word, they are even more persuasive.

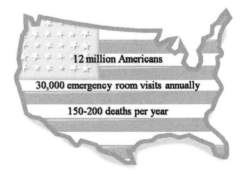

Fig. 5.3 Estimate of food allergic consumers and food allergic reactions in the United States.

The Sarah Weaver story

On August 8, 1996, my life, the lives of my husband, Robert, and two sons, and the lives of everyone in our extended family changed forever. The day before my family traveled to New York City for a late afternoon family wedding. After a brief ceremony, an elegant catered buffet was served. The food consisted of several different types of finger foods.

After a walk down the buffet line, Sarah, our 21-year-old daughter, determined that nothing appealed to her and decided to wait to stop on the way home to eat. We were going to leave in two cars. Just as we were saying our goodbyes, a woman employed by the company hosting the wedding came out of the kitchen carrying a large tray of assorted cookies. She stopped and offered cookies. Sarah asked the woman if the cookies contained any nut products. The woman serving the cookies assured her that they did not and encouraged her to help herself. Sarah took a small cookie from the tray.

A couple of minutes later, Sarah came over to me to ask if I had any Tums of Pepto Bismol with me because her stomach was upset. I told her that I did not and inquired if she was okay. She replied that she would be okay, and that she would see me at home. I kissed her goodbye and told her to be careful and that I loved her.

After taking the elevator down to the lobby, as we were going through the doors, I noticed Sarah standing on the sidewalk, bent at the waist with her hands on her hips. I asked what was wrong and Sarah replied that she was having trouble breathing. Sarah was asthmatic so it was not unusual for her to have problems such as that. I immediately became alarmed, however, when, as Sarah dispensed asthma medication into her mouth, it came back out. Simultaneously, I noticed that the rim of her ear was tinged blue.

Something told me that this was not the usual asthma attack, that something was very, very wrong. I ran into the building and called 911. When I came back out on the street a few minutes later, I saw Sarah laying in my husband and son Brian's arms. A crowd of people had gathered around. By that time, my son Matt had been summoned downstairs. Matt had just the month before graduated from Albany College of Pharmacy and was awaiting the results of his board exams to become a licensed pharmacist.

Matt looked at Sarah, saw the swelling in her throat and the rash on her face and realized that she had gone in anaphylactic shock. He ran down the street to a local pharmacy to see if he could get epinephrine, but the pharmacy was closed. As he arrived back, the first EMS unit was arriving. Matt immediately told them that Sarah needed the epinephrine. Unfortunately, they did not have the drug available and needed to wait for a second unit to arrive. The second unit attempted to administer the drug but was unsuccessful.

Sarah never regained consciousness, and after going into cardiac arrest twice and the determination that there was no brain activity, Sarah mercifully passed away the next morning at approximately 11:45 a.m.

Sarah had always been very careful not to eat anything containing nuts...not because she thought it would ever cause her death, but because nuts always made her sick to her stomach. There had been several "incidents" over the years where Sarah had a reaction to something she ate that contained nut products, but never were we told that with each incident, the likelihood of a serious reaction increases.

The death of a child is never something a parent thinks can happen to them. My first thought in the morning is always the same..."Please, God, just let it be a nightmare...let me walk into Sarah's room and find her sleeping in her bed." We will forever carry a gaping hole in our hearts and now, even the happy times are sad. Holidays, especially Christmas, Sarah's absolute favorite, are bittersweet. Whenever I see a picture of a bride, a young mother with her new baby, or even a daughter caring for her elderly mom, I think of how much of life Sarah will miss. If not for our unfailing faith in God, the belief that Sarah is an angel in heaven (a much better place than earth!), and the confidence that we will all be together again someday, I'm not sure we would have the strength to go on each day.

Fig. 5.4 The Sarah Weaver story

> Our daughter was truly the light of our lives. Sarah loved life. After her death, many people commented on how her smile could brighten a room and her sweet, caring nature was evidence in every encounter they had with her. She had her father's unique ability to see the good in everyone, make the best of every situation, and enjoy even the simplest pleasures in life.
>
> It has been four and a half years since Sarah's death, and not a day goes by without both laughter and tears...laughing abut a memory of Sarah and crying over the tragic loss of a child who gave us so much love and had such a promising life ahead, but I often say the true tragedy would have been not to be blessed with her in our lives, even for the briefest of time.

Fig. 5.4 (continued)

Make It Risk-Based

As emphasized in the previous chapter, when considering food safety training and education as a potential solution, you need to establish priorities. Good food borne diseases surveillance data and the associated contributing factors of food borne disease can serve as the basis for rationally establishing food safety training and education priorities. After conducting an initial needs-assessment, if any tasks, practices, or behaviors which have been scientifically associated with food borne disease are determined that they can be enhanced with training and education, they should be given high priority. In other words, create food safety training and education that is risk-based.

Although this point may seem intuitive, it's not always practiced. A few years ago, I purchased and reviewed most of the major commercially available food safety training curriculums that you could buy off the shelf. I compared the content in each curriculum to determine if there was any correlation with the five major risk factors reported by the CDC to most commonly contribute to foodborne disease in retail food establishments (Olsen et al., 2000). I also looked to see if the curriculums emphasized the many preparation practices and tasks performed by employees related to these risk factors. To my surprise, between curriculums, there was little to no correlation and, in some curriculums, they spent more content on items rarely implicated in foodborne disease. What is the take home message from all of this? When conducting food safety training and education, you should make sure to place proper emphasis on those topics, tasks, and behaviors that are of greater risk or more frequently associated with foodborne diseases.

Value and Respect Diversity

In the United States, it's reported that one in four foodservice employees do not speak English as their primary language at home and this trend is expected to grow (NRA, 2006). As our global community expands, this same trend (the need to communicate with people who do not share the same primary language) is increasing in retail food establishments in many parts of the world. In order to train such a diverse workforce, it's important that we as a food safety community continue to look for creative ways to enhance the training and education process.

One simple way to do this is to train and educate employees in their native language. Some may argue that in the United States, all employees should be trained in English, since generally employees are required to speak the language. To this I caution, although an employee may speak basic conversational English such as being able to say "yes sir" or "thank you", they may not have enough mastery of the language to understand some of the more complex safety processes that we as food safety professionals might try to teach them. For example, envision trying to teach an employee the requirement to cool foods from 140 to 70 F in two hours and then from 70 to 41 F in an additional 4 hours, when they do not really understand the language. This could be a very difficult thing to do. For this reason, I advocate teaching employees in their native language, within reason, for the more common languages spoken by employees in the retail food workforce.

Another way to enhance the training and education process for employees who do not speak English as their primary language is to make food safety thoughts and concepts visible through pictures, icons, and drawings. There's no doubt that visualization accelerates learning and facilitates the communication process, especially for those who do not speak our same language. So, when developing food safety training and education materials for a diverse workforce, make sure to make it visual.

Keep It Simple and User Friendly

Ralph Waldo Emerson once said, "The man who can make hard things easy is the educator." When it comes to food safety training and education, I believe this point is certainly true. The true food safety educator should be able to take a complex scientific truth about food safety and make it simple. In other words, they should be able to take a complex scientific truth and make it easy to understand, apply, and remember.

When developing training programs and designing work procedures, you should strive to keep things simple and short. Complex concepts or tasks are less likely to be understood or followed. When a concept is presented in a complex manner, employees might have a hard time following along and truly understanding what is being taught. In addition, if a procedure is too complicated, employees might be tempted to take shortcuts when performing them. Also, remember that sometimes less can be more if done effectively. Fight the temptation to be fixated on how long the training class should be. Instead, focus on delivering content in an efficient, effective, and simple manner. I believe this point – making training classes too long – is one of the biggest mistakes made by food safety educators. The teenage and adult learner's attention span is limited and, if you make the class too long and boring, you'll loose them. Focus on content, simplicity, and efficiency – not more time.

As stated previously, enhance the training and education process by making concepts visible through pictures, icons, and drawings. Learning experts know that visualization accelerates learning and facilitates communication. That's why we've all heard of the phrase, *a picture is worth a thousand words*.

Educators should also use methods that appeal to the other senses, such as hearing, smell, taste, touch, and not just sight. Research has shown that verbal or written instruction is more effective when it is combined by methods that stimulate two or more of the other senses (OSHA, 1996).

Lastly, to help with converting food safety concepts and ideas from words into images, the educator should also strive to make the education and training process participatory and hands-on. As stated in an ancient Chinese proverb, *I hear and I forget. I see and I remember. I do and I understand.* Engage employees in the learning process and they'll be much more likely to comprehend and remember what you're trying to teach them.

In closing, although this chapter was not intended to be a compressive review of education and training strategies or principles, the concepts highlighted in this chapter should be considered when evaluating the role of education and training in a behavior-based food safety management system. But education and training alone will not necessarily change the behavior of employees. Remember, education and training is only one of a series of interactive components of a behavior-based food safety management system. The next component of a behavior-based food safety management system that we will review is *communication*.

Key Points

- When trying to achieve a particular set of desired food safety related behaviors, food safety professionals often turn to training as the solution. However, it's important to realize that training in and of itself does not change behavior.
- It's important to understand that food safety training and food safety education are different – and that you need to do both.
- Food safety education generally involves the transfer of information related to food safety such as foodborne hazards, regulatory standards, and company policies to a group of individuals or employees.
- Food safety training, in contrast, involves teaching employees the details of tasks or duties assigned to them through demonstration and how they must do them to keep foods safe or make them safe.
- Behavior change is complex, so when designing food safety training and education materials, design it in a persuasive manner with behavior changes in mind.
- Employees need to understand that when it comes to food safety, there are *real risks with real consequences*.

- Personal testimonials or individual case studies are much more persuasive than group statistics.
- Make training and education risk-based by placing proper emphasis on those topics, tasks, and behaviors that are more frequently associated with foodborne diseases.
- The retail workforce continues to become more diverse. Whenever possible, convert food safety concepts and ideas from words into images.
- Keep things simple and short. Complex concepts or tasks are less likely to be understood or followed.

Chapter 6
Communicating Food Safety Effectively

> *When dealing with people, remember you are not dealing with creatures of logic, but creatures of emotion.*
>
> Dale Carnegie (1888–1955)

If you wanted to learn more about the culture of the 1940s, what would you do? Most of us would probably review newspapers, magazines, and television clips from that era. Why? Because we all know that we see, hear, and read around us every day – what we communicate – is a very good reflection of our culture. In essence, communication and culture are two sides of the same coin.

When it comes to food safety, this principle is certainly true. You can tell a lot about the food safety culture of an organization by their communication or lack of communication on the topic. If an organization is communicating about food safety and sharing information regularly with their employees about the topic, then food safety is probably an important part of their culture. It might be evident by the fact that leaders in the organization routinely talk about the importance of food safety and sanitation in meetings with their employees. You might notice it by the food safety signs or reminders you see on bulletin boards and at work stations. It might be evident by the article on food safety in the company newsletter. The bottom line is that if you're an outsider walking into this organization for the first time, there are visible demonstrations through communication that food safety is important. In contrast, even if an organization claims food safety is important, if you don't see any visible demonstrations of communication around the topic in meetings, company newsletters, signs, etc., then food safety is probably not really part of their culture. Organizations and leaders tend to talk about and communicate what is truly important to them.

The Importance of Communication

Why is communication so important? We've all heard of the saying, "the pen is mightier than the sword." That's because words have power. Words have started wars. They have helped nations make peace. They have influenced millions to take up great causes. They have made people believe in something bigger than themselves. They have sparked innovation. They have helped solved problems. Words can hurt. They can encourage. They can help educate. And very importantly, they can influence behavior.

If words are so powerful, then certainly they can be used to enhance food safety, right? For the remainder of this chapter, let's review how communication is an important component of a behavior based food safety management system and how to communicate food safety effectively.

Use a Variety of Mediums

Historically, food safety professionals have relied on a limited number of mediums to communicate food safety information. Of interest, although a variety of mediums exist to communicate food safety information, a recent study in the United Kingdom found that the most common one used by local regulatory authorities was leaflets, being used 93% of the time (Redmond & Griffith, 2006). Examples of other types of mediums available today in most companies include flyers, posters, newsletters, signs, video, company-run television channels, company intranet sites, and more. In many organizations, several of these mediums may be underutilized or not even used at all. Rather than focusing on only one or two mediums to communicate food safety information, organizations should use multiple mediums to make sure a few are actually working in reaching employees. Even if internal research data indicates that one communication vehicle, such as an internal newsletter, is the medium of choice, I always recommend redundancy. Using multiple mediums increases the chances that your food safety messages will get through and that, employees will actually see or hear them several times.

By using multiple mediums, an organization strengthens food safety as part of their culture. Let me illustrate this point. Imagine an organization that chooses to communicate food safety using a primary and favored communication vehicle, their company newsletter. The only time an employee will be reminded about food safety is if they happen to come across the newsletter and notice the article on food safety. In contrast, imagine another company that deliberately chooses to bombard their employees with "food safety sound bytes" at multiple turns. For example, when clocking in for work, they see a food safety message in the form of a sign or symbol. As they walk down the hall, they see a food safety poster on the wall. At their work station, they see visual food safety reminders related to the task or procedure at hand. When they take their break and pick up the company newsletter or listen to the company television channel, they see a piece on food safety tips, which they can apply at home. Which organization do you think will have the stronger food safety culture? You're right. In the latter organization, employees can't help but think about food safety, because it's all around them. Organizations that use multiple mediums to communicate food safety information are more likely to be successful at reaching their employees and demonstrating that food safety is an important part of their culture.

Posters, Symbols, and Slogans

Some of the most common tools used to communicate food safety messages are posters, symbols, and slogans. But are they really effective in providing instruction or influencing behavior? It depends on how they are designed and used. Behavioral research indicates that generic messages with no specific instruction concerning the desired behavior or no mention of consequences have little impact on the target behavior. With this principle in mind, it's clear that many posters, symbols, and slogans in today's workplace often miss the mark. For example, a common mistake many retail food organizations make is to post vague or unclear messages on what they expect their employees to do.

Let me provide you with four tips on making food safety posters, symbols, and slogans more effective.

Be Specific – food safety posters, symbols, and slogans should be clear and specific – not generic. Forget the cute and catchy slogans that do not describe what you want your employees to do. Although slogans such as "food safety, it's in your hands" or "think food safety" may sound catchy, they're not very effective. What do they mean? It doesn't tell an employee what it is that they must do to keep food safe. Ideally, food safety messages should be objective, observable, and related to a specific task, standard, or behavior you want your employees to do or avoid.

Placement – specific messages work best when they not only tell employees what behavior is needed, but also where the behavior is needed, such as a "don't work if you're ill" message near a time clock or a "no bare hand contact" message near a food preparation counter. To illustrate this point using a non-food safety example, imagine seeing a "slippery when wet" sign on the floor, but it wasn't near the slippery or wet condition. Do you think it would be very effective? Placement is important with food safety messages too.

Keep It Simple – avoid overly complex signs, symbols, or posters with too many messages, words, or pictures. Simplicity is best. Whenever possible, try to limit the message to one behavior to do or avoid. In this complex world we live in, there's a lot of competition for our attention. Messages that are too complex for us to quickly understand are unlikely to get our attention and will probably be overlooked.

Change It – occasionally, the messages will have to be modified or changed. The same message in the same place over a long period of time will eventually blend into the background and employees will no longer notice it unless they are new to the organization. They'll become desensitized to it. Accordingly, occasionally, you'll have to mix things up and introduce new signs, symbols, and posters to continue to get their attention.

Use More than Words

As mentioned in the previous chapter, in the coming years, it's predicted that the foodservice industry in the United States will continue to see an increase in the number of employees who do not speak English as their primary language

(NRA, 2006). And as our global community expands, this same trend (the need to communicate with people who do not share the same primary language) is increasing in many parts of the world.

Effectively communicating with individuals who do not speak English as their primary language is critical. One way to do this is to make thoughts or concepts visible through drawings, because visualization can facilitate the communication process. In fact, that's why we've all heard of the saying, "a picture is worth a thousand words."

If you think about it, the use of simple drawings or pictures to communicate with others is well-documented throughout human history. It's estimated that as early as 50,000 BC pictures first appeared as paintings or carvings in caves for communication purposes. Today, standardized drawings, better known as symbols or icons, remain important tools for communication in settings where you expect to find individuals from different cultural backgrounds, such as Olympic Games, international airports, in theme parks, and on traffic signs.

So, can standardized symbols or icons be used to communicate food safety information? Of course they can. As stated by Walt Disney years ago, "Of all of our inventions for mass communication, pictures still speak the most universally understood language." Accordingly, in 2002, under the auspices of the International Association for Food Protection's Retail Food Safety & Quality Professional Development Group, a task force developed and focus group tested a set of International Food Safety Icons as shown in Fig. 6.1. International Food Safety Icons are simple pictorial representations of important food safety tasks that can be recognized and understood regardless of a person's native language.

Although the task force did not prescribe their intended use or application, the set of International Food Safety Icons are effective visual aids, which can be used to communicate important food safety concepts in food safety training materials, as signs or reminders at food and beverage workstations, on food preparation and storage equipment, on recipe cards, or on food packages.

When communicating food safety, remember that pictures can sometimes speak louder and more effectively than words.

Have Conversations

When you think about creating a food safety communication plan, do you simply think about ways to communicate to employees or do you look for ways to let leaders, managers, and professionals on your team have food safety conversations with them? Talking to employees is very different than having food safety conversations with them. Conversations can help break down barriers and improve understanding. To illustrate this point, think for a moment about your most effective teacher or coach. Did they simply talk to you (or should I say at you), or did they have conversations with you? If you're like me, your most effective teachers and coaches had interpersonal conversations with you.

6 Communicating Food Safety Effectively

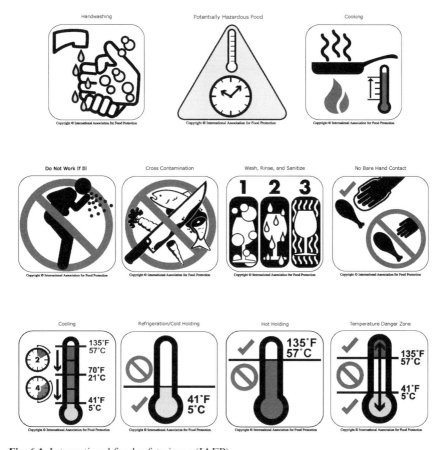

Fig. 6.1 International food safety icons (IAFP)

Let me summarize three good reasons why food safety conversations are important.

First, food safety conversations are important because they increase the likelihood that the message will be understood. Think about it, when you have an important message to deliver, do you do it with a note or pamphlet? Of course not. You do it in person because you want to make sure it's properly understood. Second, food safety conversations are important because they are participatory and not one-sided. By having a conversation about food safety with employees, you can hear from them on issues of concern, their questions, and thoughts about food safety. In other words, you can listen to them and not be the one doing all of the talking. Lastly, food safety conversations are important because they can help breakdown barriers and increase interpersonal connectedness – a critical part of shaping culture.

Ask Questions

When you think about developing a food safety communication plan, does a component of your plan include listening to your employees or does it simply include what you want to share with them? We've all heard it said that communication is a two-way street – talking and listening. One of the best ways to listen and learn is to ask questions. As stated by Dorothy Leeds (2000) in her book *The 7 Powers of Questions: Secrets to Successful Communication in Life and at Work*, "Every time you open your mouth to speak you have two options: make a statement or ask a question."

From a food safety perspective, why is it important to ask questions? Although there are several good reasons, let me summarize two important ones. First, by asking questions as part of your food safety communication plan, you may uncover potential problems or opportunities. Your employees may have challenges with meeting or complying with food safety standards that you are not aware of. By asking questions and engaging them in a conversation, you may uncover them. Second, by asking questions as part of your food safety communication plan, you make employees feel that, what they think and believe is important. Your food safety program won't be effective until you engage everyone involved in the production and service of food. When you engage your employees and make them part of the solution, you help shape and strengthen your food safety culture.

Opportunities to ask smart questions abound. For example, food safety professionals should ask smart questions when they're conducting food safety audits or inspections. If a certain standard or behavior is not being followed, rather than simply noting it on the inspection form, asking questions to understand – why? – can lead to a coaching or teaching opportunity. The types of questions asked should not be "gotcha" questions to catch someone doing something wrong. Instead, they should be genuinely inquisitive to understand the problem, so they can help with a solution. Food safety educators should ask questions when they're conducting training classes. By asking questions, they can ensure that students in the class understand the material and they also make the training more participatory. Leaders and managers within the organization should ask questions related to food safety in meetings or when walking around. And last but not least, occasionally you may want to ask questions in the form of a written, quantitative survey to measure the strength of your food safety culture (Fig. 6.2). In this manner, you can engage all of your employees and quantitatively measure changes in the strength of your food safety culture over time.

What we communicate about food safety and how we communicate it is critical. Make sure to take the time to put the right thought and effort into this important element of a behavior-based food safety management system. If you don't, you won't be effective at shaping and influencing the behaviors of your employees and the culture within your organization.

Next, let's consider the role of goals and measurements in improving food safety, the next steps in a behavior-based food safety management system.

> Rate on a 1 to 5 scale (1 = highly disagree, 5 = highly agree)
>
> 1. New employees receive food safety training before working
> 2. I have received adequate food safety training to do my job well
> 3. Food safety rules and procedures are regularly reviewed with employees
> 4. My manager coaches me on food safety practices
> 5. Employee suggestions regarding food safety are acted upon
> 6. Food safety rules and procedures are followed by employees
> 7. HACCP checks are conducted regularly in my department
> 8. Our standards and practices do not change when the health department arrives
> 9. Food safety inspections are taken seriously

Fig. 6.2 Example of a food safety culture survey questionnaire

Key Points

- You can tell a lot about the food safety culture of an organization by their communication or lack of communication on the topic.
- Words have power. Words have started wars. They have helped nations make peace. They have influenced millions to take up great causes. And so, we should realize that words can influence food safety behavior.
- Using multiple mediums to communicate food safety information increases the likelihood of reaching employees and demonstrating that food safety is an important part of the organization's culture.
- Food safety posters, signs, and symbols often miss the mark. To be effective, they should be simple, communicate what the desired behavior is, be placed where the desired behavior should occur, and changed often enough to prevent desensitizing.
- Use more than words. In the coming years, it's predicted that the foodservice industry will continue to see an increase in the need to communicate with people who do not share the same primary language. One way to do this is to make food safety thoughts or concepts visible through pictures and drawings.
- Go beyond simply talking to your employees about food safety. Have food safety conversations with them. Conversations are participatory and not one-sided. They also allow you to hear employee concerns, questions, and thoughts about food safety.
- Part of your food safety communication plan should include asking questions. By asking questions, you may uncover potential problems or opportunities that you are not aware of and you will engage your employees and make them part of the solution.

Chapter 7
Developing Food Safety Goals and Measurements

> *Man is a goal seeking animal. His life only has meaning if he is reaching out and striving for his goals.*
>
> Aristotle (384 BC–322 BC)

All meaningful progress begins with simple goal setting. For example, it may begin with the idea that we can do something better. We identify a condition that we want to improve or achieve and then we set a plan of action to get there. We measure along the way to monitor our progress and we readjust as necessary. There is no question about it; setting goals and measuring performance against those goals are critical components of the continuous improvement process.

But goals and measurements are not enough. It would be overly simplistic to think that by simply setting a goal or establishing a measurement system, things will automatically get better. Think about the many goals you have seen established – at work or at home – that have not been achieved. Why is that? Because goals and measurement systems in and of themselves are not enough to improve performance. Have you ever made a New Year's resolution? It's a goal, but the resolution itself didn't make things better or cause improvement. Surely, many of us have heard of or experienced a failed New Year's resolution. Or think about a measurement system that you might be aware of that doesn't necessarily influence behavior or progress. How about individuals on a weight loss program who weigh themselves on a scale every week, but don't experience any weight loss? Why is that? Because the act of measuring their weight on a weekly basis doesn't guarantee success.

Setting goals and measuring performance against those goals are critical components and the next step in creating a behavior-based food safety management system, but they have to be done and used correctly to be effective. Therefore, let's review several important points you should consider when developing and using food safety goals and measurement systems to enhance your organization's performance.

The Importance of Food Safety Goal Setting

The primary purpose of establishing goals is to improve performance and deliver results. When goals are established and used correctly, performance gains can be significant. For example, in documented studies, the proper use of

Fig. 7.1 ABC model

Antecedent: Behavior ⟶ Consequence

goals has led to performance gains of up to 75 percent (Pritchard, Jones, & Roth, 1988). Although these studies are unrelated to food safety, these principles hold true. Goals can improve food safety performance, increase compliance, and decrease the risk of foodborne disease.

Goals are effective, because when they are established properly, they are powerful antecedents to desired performance or behavior. An antecedent is anything that comes before a behavior that contains information about behavioral consequences (Daniels & Daniels, 2004). Accordingly, goals alone will not result in improved performance unless they are consistently paired with consequences. This approach to how to establish and use goals is based on the ABC Model developed through scientific research in the field of behavioral analysis (Fig. 7.1). Imagine setting a goal that would require a group of employees to work hard to meet it, yet if they did, there would be no positive consequence for them. They wouldn't be recognized for their accomplishment or they wouldn't be rewarded for their achievement. Do you think the goal would be very effective in motivating the employees? Of course not. When establishing food safety goals, you should always pair them with consequences.

Establishing Effective Food Safety Goals

Many organizations and companies have their own approaches to goal setting. However, we have all heard of goals that were not attained. Although there may be valid reasons, one of the most common reasons for not reaching goals is that the goal itself was poorly developed. Let me summarize five important things to consider when establishing food safety goals.

Make Them Achievable – one of the most common mistakes made when developing goals is to set them too high. Sure, I know, we've all heard of the term "stretch goals." I, too, believe that goals should be set high, but not too high where they are unachievable. Setting unachievable goals can do more harm than good. If employees feel a goal is too high, they may not even try to reach it, because they feel it's unattainable. In other words, employees may simply give up and not even try to do what you're asking them to do. Goals should be set high but achievable. And needless to say, the goal must be under the person or work team's control.

Be Specific – goals that are too vague or generic are useless. For example, establishing a goal that you will improve food safety this year is meaningless to most employees. It doesn't tell them what it is that you want them to do or get better at. A better goal might be to state that you want to improve internal food safety audits scores by a certain percentage during the next fiscal year. Ideally or even better yet, goals should be targeted to very specific behaviors or conditions you want to improve. For example, a goal might be that you want to reduce the frequency of an organization's most frequent violation or risk factor by 20 percent. More specifically, you might state that you want to see an increase in a specific desired behavior, such as hand washing when needed, and state it in quantitative terms.

Make Them Risk-Based – in a retail food establishment or organization, there might be the temptation to want to create goals to improve performance in many areas. Focus your food safety goal setting on those conditions or behaviors that have been scientifically associated with food borne disease. In other words, create food safety goals that are risk-based and, if achieved, will further reduce the likelihood of food borne disease. Food borne diseases surveillance data, published reports on contributing factors of food borne disease, and internal audit findings should serve as useful information to help you with food safety goal setting.

Make Them Measurable – goals that cannot be quantitatively measured are not useful in improving performance. Without measurements, the interpretation on whether or not a goal is being achieved is subject to bias. When establishing a food safety goal related to a specific behavior or condition, if you don't have a measurement system already in place to track progress, create one.

Write Them Down – it's been said that goals that are not written down are just wishes. Food safety goals should be clearly documented, in quantitative terms, and shared with those who share in the responsibility of achieving them. Progress toward meeting the goal should be monitored frequently and specific performance feedback given along the way.

Why Measure Food Safety?

Without measurement, you cannot improve food safety performance or further reduce the risk of food borne disease. It is only through the use of measurements that you can know if your organization's food safety performance is getter better, staying the same, or getting worse.

Edwards Deming once said, "You can't manage what you don't measure." Although this point is true, it is only true if you use the measurement to manage performance. Equally important to the measurement itself and maybe more difficult to do is how to use the results of measurements to improve food safety performance. I suggest that taking the measurement itself might be the easier part of what we do and it's what most food safety professionals are taught to do. Using the measurement to strengthen or manage performance is more difficult and most food safety professionals do not receive adequate education and training in this area. For example, as food safety professionals, we receive training on how to conduct an audit or perform certain microbiological tests. We often compare audits to see if we're measuring the same things or are asking the same questions. We rarely talk about what we do with the results of food safety measurements or how we use them to achieve a desired goal.

Think about organizations that you might know of or have heard about, including regulatory agencies, which have conducted and accumulated enormous amounts of measurements over the years. Some agencies and organizations have literally taken and recorded thousands of food safety measurements on paper or in a data base, yet they have not made maximum use of them, nor have they seen proportionately enhanced performance as a result of the numerous measurements they have taken.

Let me share a few tips on how to maximize the use of food safety measurements.

Use Them to Catch People Doing Things Right – food safety measurements conducted by food safety professionals in retail have been historically used to catch people doing things wrong or detect conditions that do not meet a certain standard. Remember, when developing a behavior-based food safety management, you have to think differently. You need to think about all that you do, including measurements, in terms of human behavior and motivation. Food safety measurements should, first and foremost, be conducted to catch people doing things right – not catch them doing things wrong. Sure, if a food safety measurement reveals a behavior or condition is not up to standard, it has to be dealt with and corrected, but don't miss an opportunity to provide positive reinforcement for behaviors and conditions that are right.

Use Them to Trend and Compare – as stated earlier, without measurement, you cannot improve food safety performance or further reduce the risk of food borne disease. Use measurements to determine if your organization's food safety performance is getting better, staying the same, or getting worse. For example, you can compare specific risk factor rates from audits or HACCP checks that you're concerned about from month to month, year to year, and over time. This information can help you identify those specific issues that have not progressed at the rate desired and allow you to target intervention measures for improvement. You can also compare performance between establishments and determine if certain stores are performing better than others. This approach, with proper reporting, can also lead to friendly competition and better performance. In addition, with proper use of information technology systems to capture measurements, you can create more rapid surveillance and data-mining abilities that will identify opportunities in almost real-time and allow you to respond more quickly to specific issues of concern or performance headed in the wrong direction.

Use Them to Innovate – even if your organization has made great progress in improving its food safety performance, it can get better if it uses it's measurements to reveal areas of opportunity and create innovative solutions to solving them. A simple definition of an innovation is the act of introducing something new. From a food safety perspective, an innovation can be a new or safer way of performing a certain food production task. It can be the use of a new food safety product or a new approach to a particularly challenging situation. The bottom line is that an innovation leads to a proactive change and a proactive change can lead to even greater food safety performance. Use food safety measurements to identify areas of opportunity and then analyze those areas intensely to determine the root causes to the issues. For example, if an organization's data tells them that they detect employees repeatedly using unsafe practices that can lead to cross-contamination in a particular work station, the solution may not be retraining. Upon closer examination, the solution may be to redesign the work flow at the station or the station itself. Remember, use food safety measurements to innovate, because without innovation and change, there can be no progress.

What Should You Measure?

In the field of retail food safety, historically, there has been an over-reliance on measuring physical conditions of the establishment and food. For example, a typical retail food safety inspection will involve auditing the temperature of cold foods, hot foods, and the cooking and cooling of foods. It most likely will also include visual observations for the cleanliness of the facility and surfaces, such as cutting boards, food equipment, and food preparation areas. Clearly, all of these are important. However, historically, retail food safety inspections have been overly focused on the physical conditions of the establishment – not behaviors or processes. Physical attributes of the establishment and the food only provide a brief snapshot of the food safety risk and performance of an establishment. Studies by Jones et al. (2004) and Mullen et al. (2002) have suggested that there is no correlation with retail food safety inspection scores and the likelihood that an establishment might be involved in an outbreak.

To thoroughly evaluate the food safety risk and performance of a retail establishment, you need to do more than simply measure the physical condition of the establishment and the food. Ideally, you should also measure other factors related to human behavior and organizational culture that are critical for food safety success.

Below are three other critical items that should be measured to thoroughly assess the food safety risk and performance of retail food establishments.

Measure Processes – measuring end states is not good enough. You need to measure the process too. If the end state of a physical condition, such as the temperature of a food product is acceptable, it doesn't tell you if the results were achieved because of a good production process or by mere chance. It also doesn't tell you if the results are consistently achievable. The acceptable end state condition doesn't paint the whole picture. Dr Edwards Deming taught us this principle all too well. It is more important to inspect and test the process than it is the finished product or desired end state. To illustrate this point, imagine a car manufacturer that doesn't test their manufacturing process.

They only inspect the quality of completed cars coming off of their manufacturing line. Do you think they will consistently manufacture high quality automobiles? Of course not. This point is true in food production too. To truly understand if food can be made safely on a consistent basis, inspect the production process – not just the finished product. Clearly, this will require more time than a traditional end-point inspection and it will require an understanding of the production process. If the production processes is thoroughly understood, one way to do this is to measure certain critical points or steps in the preparation method to make sure they are being properly followed and conducted.

Measure Knowledge – in the field of retail food safety, the measurement of knowledge is largely achieved through the requirement for chefs or managers in charge of retail establishments to become certified food safety professionals by passing regulatory and industry recognized exams. There is a growing body of evidence that suggests that retail establishments with certified managers are less likely to experience a food borne outbreak (Hedberg et al., 2006). Although this is great, having a certified food manager on-board in the establishment it is not the only way to measure knowledge. Knowledge assessments and measurements can be built into the retail food safety audit or inspection itself. And it doesn't have to be limited to the manager or chef in-charge; it can involve front-line employees too. For example, if a full-service restaurant chain trains it's front line employees to make sure to get a chef or manager in charge if a customer has any food allergy questions, then during a retail food safety audit, front line employees can be asked, what do you do if a customer informs you they have a food allergy? Measuring knowledge to see if employees actually know and remember what they have been trained to do not only gives confidence that the employees have learned what is expected of them, it also helps to re-emphasize certain key points.

Measure Behavior – it has been said, what we know is of little consequence. It's what we do that is important. It's one thing to measure knowledge, but do employees actually do what they are expected and trained to do? The only way to know for sure is to measure specific behaviors or activities. Measuring behaviors and activities can be difficult and time consuming. However, if there are certain behaviors or activities that you want to make sure are being properly conducted, then after the expectations have been clearly communicated and training has been provided, they should be occasionally observed and measured to determine if they are being done consistently and correctly.

Lagging Versus Leading Indicators of Food Safety

As a field, food safety professionals have relied mainly on outcome-based measures (*lagging indictors*) to determine if we are making progress in the battle against foodborne disease. For example, as illustrated in Fig. 7.2, foodborne

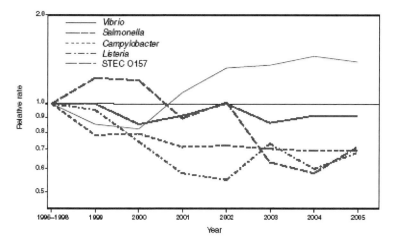

Fig. 7.2 Relative rates of laboratory-diagnosed cases of foodborne infections in the United States. (Foodborne disease active surveillance network, 1996–2005)

disease surveillance data or measures allow us to determine what the incidence rate of illnesses due to certain pathogens are from year to year (CDC, 2006). Foodborne disease surveillance is the ultimate measure to determine if progress is being made in reducing food borne illness. Another outcome-based measure obtained through microbiological baseline surveys is the prevalence of certain foodborne pathogens in the food supply (USDA, 2006). This type of information, data on pathogens in foods, allows us to understand exposure of consumers to certain foodborne pathogens by food product type. When interpreted over time, microbiological baseline measures are useful for evaluating the effectiveness of intervention strategies on reducing microbial contamination (Fig. 7.3).

Although such outcome-based measures are critically important and extremely useful to observe trends and establish priorities, as risk managers we know that to achieve reductions in foodborne disease incidence rates or microbial

Y 2005

Product	Baseline Prevalence (%)	Large		Small		Very Small		Unknown		All Sizes	
		# Sample	% Positive	# Sample	% Positive	# Sample	% Positive	# Sample	% Positive	# Sample	% Positive
Broilers	20.0	6,853	14.7%	2,458	18.6%	280	32.9%	1	0.0%	9,592	16.3%
Market Hogs	8.7	1,410	2.2%	1,750	5.2%	3,488	3.6%	0		6,648	3.7%
Cows/Bulls	2.7	229	0.0%	975	1.5%	745	1.5%	0		1,949	1.3%
Steers/Heifers	1.0	788	0.0%	552	0.9%	750	0.9%	0		2,090	0.6%
Ground Beef	7.5	544	2.2%	9,070	1.4%	9,751	0.8%	0		19,365	1.1%
Ground Chicken	44.6	0		133	33.1%	12	25.0%	0		145	32.4%
Ground Turkey	49.9	799	24.8%	86	14.0%	40	12.5%	0		925	23.2%

Fig. 7.3 Percent positive *salmonella* tests in the HACCP verification testing program by product class and calendar year, 2005

contamination rates, we need to implement effective food safety management processes and we need to change behaviors (*leading indicators*). Understanding outcome-based foodborne disease statistics or measures, the lagging indicators, is very important, but they are not enough. We need to be equally or even more focused on the processes or behaviors – the leading indicators of food safety – that can result in lower rates of illnesses. To do this, we need to clearly understand that relationship between the two measures (lagging and leading indicators) and we need to proactively create and manage leading measures of food safety.

To illustrate this point using a simple analogy, let's consider a person's desire to lose weight. The ultimate measure of whether or not the person is experiencing success is the outcome-based measure, the lagging indicator, of the person's actual weight as measured on the scale each week. But to manage weight loss, the person would need leading indicators too, not just an outcome-based measure, to help them stay on the right track. For example, the person would likely count their daily caloric intake – a leading measure. They might also count the number of calories burned or time devoted to exercise. The bottom line is that to be successful, the person would need to manage the leading indicators of weight loss. This point or concept is certainly true in the field of food safety too.

No single leading indicator or measure will be fully adequate to manage food safety risk within a complex retail food establishment. Instead, a range of food safety measures should be considered to manage and improve food safety performance (Fig. 7.4). They can range from quantitative and qualitative measures to assess employee knowledge and attitudes about food safety to very specific observations of behaviors identified as contributing factors of foodborne disease. Leading indicators can include HACCP checks or measures of critical control points to make sure they're within critical limits and the results of internal and regulatory food safety audits of specific risk factors identified as important causes of foodborne outbreaks in retail food settings

Lagging Indicators	Leading Indicators
Foodborne Disease Surveillance Data	Quantitative & Qualitative Culture Surveys
Microbiological Baseline Surveys	Knowledge Assessments
Food Recalls	Behavioral Observations
	HACCP Checks and Measurements
	Audits of Risk Factors
	Microbial Validations

Fig. 7.4 Leading versus lagging indicators (measures) of food safety

(FDA Retail Food Program Steering Committee, 2000). The bottom line is that to proactively manage food safety risk and performance, risk managers need more than lagging indicators of food safety. They need to create and manage leading indicators too.

Remember, goals and measurements are an important component of a behavior-based food safety management system, but they will not result in consistently improved performance unless they are consistently paired with consequences. This is the next step in creating a behavior-based food safety management system.

Key Points

- All meaningful progress begins with simple goal setting.
- Goals are effective, because when they are established properly, they are powerful antecedents to desired performance or behavior.
- An antecedent is anything that comes before a behavior that contains information about behavioral consequences. Accordingly, goals alone will not result in improved performance unless they are consistently paired with consequences.
- When establishing food safety goals, make them *achievable, specific, risk-based*, and *measurable*. Also, make sure to *write them down*.
- Only through the use of valid measurements can you know if your organization's food safety performance is getting better, staying the same, or getting worse.
- Use food safety measurements to (a) *Catch People Doing Things Right*, (b) *Trend and Compare*, and (c) *Innovate*.
- To evaluate food safety performance, you need to do more than simply measure the physical condition of the establishment and the food. You should also measure factors such as *processes, knowledge,* and, most importantly, *behavior*.
- No single measure will be fully adequate to manage food safety risk in a complex retail establishment. Therefore, use a combination of both *leading* and *lagging* indicators to gauge performance.
- To be effective in improving performance, remember that food safety goals and measurements must be consistently paired with consequences.

Chapter 8
Using Consequences to Increase or Decrease Behaviors

> *The consequence of an act affects the probability of it occurring again.*
>
> B.F. Skinner (1904–1990)

At the end of the day, what a group of employees or individuals know about food safety principles or what they think or believe about food safety is of less importance. It's what they do – their behaviors – that is critically important. So how can we help shape or reinforce proper food safety behaviors? Well, I believe one of the most important ways is through the proper use of consequences. That's right – consequences.

As I have stated before, the words we use and how we use them are important. So let's take a moment to review the word *consequence*. The word consequence is often interpreted to have a negative connotation. Most people believe that a consequence is something negative or bad. But consequences can be negative and they can also be positive.

So what is a consequence? According to Webster's dictionary (1985), *a consequence is something produced by a cause or necessarily following from a set of conditions; important with respect to power to produce an effect.*

Why are consequences important? Well, if you agree with Webster's definition above, consequences are important because they increase or decrease the likelihood of behavior occurring again. Every single day, people do things because of consequences or potential consequences. Yes, the consequences of an act affect the probability of it occurring again. If we do something that produces a consequence that we like or that benefits us, let's say we get recognized or rewarded for the behavior; we are more likely to do it again. If we do something that produces a consequence that we don't like or that does not benefit us, for example it produces discomfort; we are less likely to do it again. According to Daniels (1999), *behavioral consequences are those things and events that follow a behavior and change the probability that the behavior will be repeated in the future.*

If consequences help increase or decrease behaviors, then certainly they can be used to enhance food safety performance, right? Of course they can. Remember, food safety performance is a result of behaviors. If an organization is not seeing improvements in food safety, then one contributing factor may be that they are not effectively using consequences to manage performance. Organizations that are able to meet specific and objective food safety goals year after year and improve food safety performance most likely have figured out a way to develop effective consequences. Those that do not are not properly using consequences to their advantage. Creating and utilizing effective consequences is the next step in a behavior based food safety management system.

Determine the Cause of Performance Problems

In the last chapter, I mentioned that an antecedent is anything that comes before a behavior that contains information about behavioral consequences. Antecedents provide proper motivation to get us to try a behavior. Consequences affect the probability that the behavior will occur again.

However, before you start using consequences to start managing food safety performance, you should determine why you are not seeing the desired behavior or why you are seeing the undesired behavior. In other words, a thorough needs-assessment should be performed. You should determine if the performance problem is a *lack of skill* (the employee doesn't know what to do or know how to do it), a result of an *ineffective system* or work set-up that leads to difficulty in performing the desired behavior (wrong equipment, wrong work tools, or poor lay-out), or a *lack of motivation* (the employee simply doesn't want to do it or doesn't like doing it).

Let me summarize these three performance problems below.

Lack of Skill – problems due to a lack of skill can be addressed by making sure performance expectations are clear and the employee is trained and educated on the specific task or behavior of concern. As reported by Fournies (1999), the most common reason managers give as to why employees at work don't do what they are supposed to do is, "they don't know what they are supposed to do." Make sure that the employee knows what to do and that they have the skills necessary to do the job.

Ineffective System – if a particular outcome or behavior is not being achieved and you know with certainty that the employee has the right skill set, examine the system before you jump to a conclusion that the employee lacks motivation. Is the work-system set up for success? Does the employee have the right work tools or equipment to get the job done effectively? Is the work-flow designed in a manner to minimize taking shortcuts or developing a work-around because of an inefficient design? For example, if the undesired behavior of cross-contamination is observed with an employee working at a ready to eat sandwich station as well as assisting with the handling raw animal proteins, before you jump to the erroneous conclusion that it's a lack of motivation, ask a few critical questions. Is the work station designed in manner to minimize cross-contamination? Do the employees have adequate time in between tasks to wash their hands? Are they provided with the right work tools to minimize the potential for cross-contamination? Sometimes, deviations from the desired behavior are not a result of lack of skill or knowledge. Instead, the deviation is due to an ineffective system that encourages shortcuts or workaround.

Lack of Motivation – the absence or inconsistent demonstration of the desired behavior or the observance of the undesired behavior could be due to a lack of motivation. If the employee has the appropriate skills to perform the task correctly and the work-system is designed well, but the employee still demonstrates the undesired behavior, they may simply lack the motivation. In this scenario, the appropriate use of consequences is likely to help with managing performance. Remember, the effective use of consequences will affect the probability of the desired or undesired behavior occurring again.

Creating Consequences for Food Safety

According to behavioral scientists, there are four types of behavioral consequences that an organization can use to get results. *Positive reinforcement* and *negative reinforcement* are two behavioral consequences that increase the probability of a behavior occurring again. *Punishment* and *penalty* are two behavioral consequences that decrease behavior (Fig. 8.1).

For the purpose of our discussion on this topic, I will simplify consequences and call them either positive or negative. Positive consequences are consequences that increase the likelihood of the behavior occurring again. Negative consequences generally decrease the likelihood of the behavior or, alternatively, are viewed as useful in trying to sustain certain desired behaviors out of fear of receiving a negative consequence. For example, a person driving might choose to follow the speed limit (desired behavior) and not speed (undesired behavior) out of concern of receiving a speeding ticket (negative consequence).

Behavioral scientists report that immediate and certain consequences are more effective at influencing behavior than consequences that are delayed or uncertain. Although we won't spend much time on this important principle in this book, you should be aware of this very critical point. To illustrate, let me provide a simple example. If an employee knows that when frying fish in a fryer, they rush or are careless, they are more likely to splatter oil and receive a painful burn, they will probably use care, not rush, and follow the proper procedure. The naturally occurring negative consequence, in this case the likelihood of receiving a painful burn, is fairly certain and immediate. In contrast, if the consequence is uncertain, it is less likely to influence behavior.

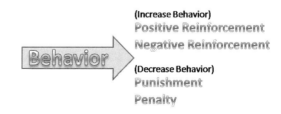

Fig. 8.1 The effects of positive and negative consequences on behavior

Lastly, be aware that there are natural occurring consequences and management-created consequences. The example used above where an employee is more likely to get burned if they rush and do not follow procedures is a naturally occurring consequence. Management-created consequences do not occur naturally. They only happen because a manager causes them to. They require consistent management observation, commitment, and follow through. For example, if when an employee meets a certain performance objective or demonstrates a certain behavior, the manager gives them a small reward and thanks them, this is an intentionally created positive consequence.

In summary and simply put, there are two important tools an organization can use to enhance food safety performance. One is the development and use of positive consequences for food safety and, the other, is the creation and use of negative consequences. If your organization does not have a clear strategy on how to use positive consequences to enhance food safety and a clear and documented policy on how to issue negative consequences, then may I suggest that you are probably not using consequences to their maximum potential.

Positive Consequences

Positive consequences can occur naturally or they can be created. Often times, naturally occurring positive food safety consequences are not obvious and, in fact, following proper food safety requirements may affect the performer, the employee, negatively. While the worker may understand that following the proper food safety procedure or behavior ultimately benefits the customer, because it reduces the risk of foodborne disease (a positive consequence), the immediate consequence to the worker might not be so obvious. In fact, for the worker, following the proper procedure or displaying the proper behavior might be perceived as penalty to them by causing them a little more effort or time. In these situations, it is important for the leaders of the organization to point out and help employees appreciate the naturally occurring positive consequence as well as create more certain positive consequences to manage food safety performance and increase the likelihood of desired behaviors occurring again and again.

Again, management-created positive consequences do not occur naturally. It is these management-created positive consequences for food safety that I believe are needed to significantly enhance employee performance in food safety. Historically, as a profession, I believe food safety professionals have been focused all too often on creating negative consequences for less than optimal food safety performance. For example, food safety professionals for years have cited violations on inspection reports that get distributed to senior management. Regulatory agencies may threaten establishments with warnings and even fines. Fears of penalties and punishment have been one of the primary tools used by regulatory officials in attempt to enhance compliance. However, when food safety professionals place an overreliance on negative consequences, it demonstrates that they really do not fully understand how to utilize consequences to drive enhanced performance. Think about it, employees will not be inspired to perform to their maximum potential out of fear of being punished or receiving a negative consequence. A work environment driven by fear of negative consequences is not a very nice work environment. Although negative consequences certainly have their place in managing food safety performance, they are not the only consequences that should be used.

Although some have stated that you must have a right balance between positive consequences and negative consequences, sometimes referred to as positive and negative reinforcement, there really is no magic ratio. Rather than focusing on an exact ratio, remember this very important point. Studies have repeatedly shown that emphasis on positive consequences over negative consequences generally leads to enhanced performance and results. For example, Madesen and Madsen (1974) found that teachers who used positive reinforcement over negative at a ratio of at least 4:1 or better were able to achieve higher performance and discipline in their classrooms. There are other studies that have demonstrated this same principle. For enhanced performance and results, the frequency of positive consequences or reinforcement should significantly outweigh the use of negative consequences.

In addition to enhancing individual personal performance, positive consequences, often called reinforcement and recognition, can also be directly linked to enhanced bottom-line business results. Gostick and Elton (2007) summarized research conducted by the Jackson Organization that indicates companies that effectively manage positive consequences and reinforcement have a much higher return on equity (a measure of profitability, asset management, and financial leverage), a higher return on assets (fiscal year's assets divided by total assets), and better operating margins. Based on these findings, do you think companies that effectively manage positive consequences for food safety will perform better than those that do not? Research in other areas suggest they will.

Before beginning to use positive consequences in an effort to enhance food safety performance, a company or organization should ask itself two basic questions. The first question should be what should the organization positively reinforce? A good place to start is with what you are already measuring. Remember, you should already be using leading and lagging indicators to manage food safety performance. This would be a good place to start, since you have already deemed these things to be important. Secondly, you should ask yourself, what are the types of positive consequences or reinforcement the company should consider?

Although not expected to be a comprehensive list of potential positive consequences an organization may choose to use to enhance food safety performance, let me provide a brief summary, utilizing a layered approach, of the types of things that should be reinforced and the types of positive consequences or reinforcement a company may consider.

Specific Desired Behaviors – remember, what we know is of little importance; it's what we do that is important. If there are certain behaviors or activities that you want to make sure are being properly conducted, then make sure you occasionally observe them and reinforce them. Often times this type of approach is viewed as on-the-spot, individualized, and informal reinforcement. Ideally, it should be frequent enough, specific to desired behavior, and given in close proximity or in a timely manner immediately following the observation of the behavior itself. Different types of positive reinforcement include a simple verbal "thank you." Don't underestimate the power of a simple "thank you" for a job well done. Most employees sincerely appreciate verbal recognition by their manager or leader. Other types of positive reinforcement can range from more formal tokens of appreciation, such as a food safety recognition card or a food safety pin, to small gift certificates worth monetary value. One important key to remember is that you want to strike the right balance between creating positive consequences and recognition for a job well done versus simply recognizing employees for what they are expected to do. In summary, remember that creating positive consequences or positive reinforcement for certain desired behaviors will only lead to more of that behavior. It will also communicate to other employees that the behavior being recognized is valued by you as a leader and by the organization.

Process or Conditions – when considering the types of things to reinforce or create positive consequences for, you might want to consider processes that are being followed or conditions that are being met that exceed minimum standards. For example, if a food service kitchen repeatedly conducts all of their HACCP checks despite being short staffed and overwhelmingly busy, this might be worthy of recognition, especially if data for the organization suggests that conducting and documenting HACCP checks remains an opportunity. As yet another example, if you walk into an establishment and it is amazingly clean, well organized, and it is clear that the team is paying attention to procedural details, cleanliness and sanitation; this team might be a great candidate for positive reinforcement or recognition. Although the observation that the facility is in outstanding condition is not part of a formal inspection and will be partly subjective, it can still be positively reinforced and, if so, is likely to lead to that facility remaining in that condition for the formal inspection process and day-to-day. In this situation, positive consequences or reinforcement might be appropriate for the manager and/or the team. Positive consequences can range from a personalized congratulatory note or certificate for each team member to a party or celebration in recognition of the team's efforts in food safety and sanitation.

Outcomes – as stated earlier, without measurement, you cannot improve food safety performance or further reduce the risk of foodborne disease. Bottom line outcome measurements, such as specific reductions in risk factor violation rates or improvement in overall audit scores, will be evidence that your organization's food safety performance is getting better. Remember, performance outcomes are directly linked to specific behaviors, which you should be reinforcing. Nevertheless, you may want to still recognize the bottom line outcome or results. For example, you might want to check if specific risk factor rates from audits or HACCP checks that you're concerned about are improving from month to month, year to year, or over time. Locations that are showing significant improvement, meeting established targets or goals, or whose performance is considered best in class for the organization, should be recognized. Positive consequences or recognition can range from very formal awards given at the company's award ceremony to financial incentives in the way of bonuses or tied into the annual merit process.

In summary, creating and properly administering positive consequences for desired food safety behaviors, processes, and outcomes will lead to enhanced food safety performance. As summarized by Dr Michael LeBoeuf in his book, *The Greatest Management Principle in the World* (1985), managers don't get what they hope for, train for, beg for, or even demand. Managers get what they recognize and reward through positive consequences.

Negative Consequences

In the previous section, we have reviewed how management-created positive consequences can be used to increase the likelihood of desired behaviors occurring again. However, sometimes the behavior that is occurring is an undesired one and we want it to stop. In these situations, just like positive consequences can be used to increase the likelihood of the behavior; negative consequences can be used to decrease the likelihood of an undesired behavior from occurring again.

As mentioned previously, when negative consequences follow a behavior in attempt to decrease or stop it, these consequences are generally referred to as punishment or penalties. In fact, these two types of behavioral consequences are commonly used in society by public health and law enforcement officials in an attempt to decrease unsafe, unhealthy, or illegal behaviors. For example, if you receive a speeding ticket with a steep financial penalty after exceeding the speed limit, this is a negative consequence intended to slow you down. How about threat of prison time for certain crimes? Although negative consequences may be effective in influencing short-term behavioral change, many have questioned their ability to produce genuine, long-term behavioral change. Think about the speeding example used above. How many drivers do you think who receive a speeding ticket will actually stop speeding for a prolonged period of time? In many cases, the desired behavior (traveling under the speed limit), will only take place when there is a fear of being caught. In other words, the behavioral change is not genuine and sustained.

Although negative consequences should be used from time to time in the field of food safety, they should be used with care and discretion. Ideally, negative consequences for knowingly or intentional unsafe behaviors can be integrated into the disciplinary or performance management process already established or in place at your organization. For example, disciplinary measures can range from a simple verbal coaching discussion immediately after witnessing the unsafe behavior to, depending on how egregious is the food safety offense, more formal documented written reprimands to immediate termination.

Remember, studies have repeatedly shown that an emphasis on positive consequences over negative consequences generally leads to enhanced performance. As previously stated, an overreliance on negative consequences will not inspire employees to perform to their maximum potential, it does not bring out the best in people, and it certainly doesn't lead to a very nice work environment. Although negative consequences certainly have there place in managing food safety performance, they are not the only consequences that should be used.

In summary, as you consider the role consequences should play in your food safety efforts, remember that behavioral change is complex and that consequences are only one small component of a comprehensive behavior-based food safety management system. Consequences certainly play a critical part, but in and off themselves, they will not result in consistent and sustained behavioral change. Consequences are most effective when they are an integrated part of a comprehensive behavior-based food safety management system.

Key Points

- One of the most important ways to shape or reinforce proper food safety behaviors is through the use of consequences.
- *Consequences* are those things and events that follow a behavior and change the probability that the behavior will be repeated in the future.
- Before using consequences to influence behavior, conduct a needs-assessment and determine why the performance problem is occurring.
- Performance problems can be due to a lack of skill, a result of an ineffective system or work set-up that leads to difficulty in performing the desired behavior, or a lack of motivation.
- Consequences can be used to shape or influence performance problems due to a lack of motivation.
- Positive consequences are consequences that increase the likelihood of the behavior occurring again.
- Negative consequences generally decrease the likelihood of the behavior or, alternatively, are viewed as useful in trying to sustain certain desired behaviors out of fear of receiving a negative consequence.
- Immediate and certain consequences are more effective at influencing behavior than consequences that are delayed or uncertain.
- Positive and negative consequences can occur naturally or they can be management created. Management-created positive consequences are needed and they can significantly enhance employee performance in food safety.

8 Using Consequences to Increase or Decrease Behaviors   75

- For enhanced performance and results, the frequency of positive consequences or reinforcement should significantly outweigh the use of negative consequences.
- Consequences certainly play a critical part, but in and off themselves, they will not result in consistent and sustained behavioral change. Consequences are most effective when they are an integrated part of a comprehensive *behavior-based food safety management system.*

Chapter 9
Tying It All Together – Behavior-Based Food Safety Management

> *Good management is better than good income.*
> Portuguese Proverb

As with other chapters, I would like to begin this one by taking a moment to review two words. The first word is *behavior*. According to Webster's dictionary (1985), *behavior is the response of an individual or group to its environment.* The second word is *management*. Webster's dictionary (1985) states that *management is the judicious use of means to accomplish an end.* Combined together, behavior-based management can then be viewed as the system of management (in our case a behavior-based food safety management system), based on the sciences of human behavior and organizational culture, which is used by an organization to produce results.

Remember, fundamental principles of management, especially those related to organizational culture and behavior as defined in this book, are critical concepts that must be understood, executed, and overseen well if an organization wants to enhance their food safety performance. However, principles of managing people, ultimately translated into influencing and shaping behavior and performance, might seem simple, but they are not. They are complex. And more importantly, they are rarely integrated into approaches for enhancing food safety performance and into food safety management practices.

Throughout this book (and as illustrated in Fig. 9.1), I have attempted to provide you with a model of high level concepts related to shaping a food safety culture and creating a behavior-based food safety management system. To effectively create or sustain a food safety culture, remember that it is critical to have a systems thinking mindset. You must realize the interdependency of each of the various efforts your organization chooses to put into practice and how the totality of those efforts influences people's thoughts and behaviors.

Management or Leadership?

Having spent so much of this book on the topic of good management, I would be remiss to close without elaborating on the differences between management and leadership.

Fig. 9.1 Behavior-based food safety management system continuous improvement model

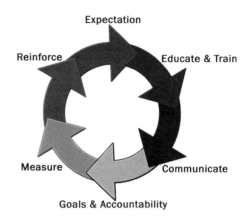

As I stated earlier in this book, it's interesting to me that in the field of food safety today, we often talk about food safety management. We rarely talk about food safety leadership. But management and leadership are different. A manager's job is to oversee and optimize organizational processes to deliver results. A leader's job is to change to process to deliver even greater results.

I should note that in today's business world, the word *management* is often implied to be inferior to the word *leadership*. Think about it. Most business books these days are about leadership. Companies talk about leadership. Politicians emphasize leadership. And there are numerous seminars and conferences on the topic of leadership. However, I do not believe that one term (*management* or *leadership*) is inferior or superior to the other. They're just different. In fact, in the field of food safety, we need both – food safety management and food safety leadership – and they are both absolutely critical to protecting public health.

To make improved reductions in the global burden of foodborne disease, we need *better* food safety management (specifically behavior based food safety management) and *more* food safety leadership. Quite frankly, creating a behavior-based food safety management system is both – food safety management and food safety leadership – because it's a new and improved way to manage food safety performance.

As a recap, let me summarize some of the key concepts presented throughout this book by contrasting a traditional food safety management approach to a *behavior-based food safety management* approach.

Traditional Food Safety Management Versus Behavior-Based Food Safety Management

As I began to write this book, I performed an interesting exercise. I did an Internet search on the term *food safety management* using my favorite search engine. As you can imagine, I came up with numerous hits. Most of the sites I came across were related to food safety management systems, food safety management programs, and food safety management certifications. There were many. However, not a single one referred to *behavior-based food safety management* as described in this book.

Below are some of the key concepts we've reviewed throughout this book on the main differences between a traditional food safety management approach versus a behavior-based food safety management approach (Fig. 9.2).

Traditional food safety management focuses on processes; behavior-based food safety management focuses on people.

The term food safety management system, as traditionally used, often refers to a system that includes having prerequisite programs in place, good manufacturing practices (GMPs), a Hazard Analysis of Critical Control Point plan, a recall procedure, and so on. It's a very process focused system. Don't get me wrong, well-defined processes and standards are critical. But as we have learned throughout this book, having well-defined processes and standards are not enough. A behavior-based food safety management system is process focused, but it's also people focused. Remember, at the end of the day, food safety equals behavior. And to improve the food safety performance of your organization, you have to change people's behaviors.

Traditional food safety management is primarily based on the food sciences; behavior-based food safety management is based on the food sciences, the behavioral sciences, and the scientific knowledge of organizational culture.

Traditional food safety managers are focused on the principles of food safety, temperature control, and sanitation – the food sciences. They believe that managing these scientific principles will lead to food safety success. Behavior-based food safety managers have mastery over the food sciences. But they understand that the food sciences are not enough. They understand that achieving food safety success requires not only an understanding of the food sciences, but of the behavioral sciences too. Accordingly, they are students of behavioral change theories, the behavioral sciences, and principles related to organizational culture.

	Traditional Food Safety Management	Behavior-based Food Safety Management
	• Focuses on processes.	• Focuses on processes and people.
	• Primarily based on Food Science.	• Based on Food Science, Behavioral Science, and Organizational Culture.
	• Simplistic view of behavior change	• Behavior change is complex.
	• Linear cause and effect thinking.	• Systems thinking.
	• Creates a Food Safety Program.	• Creates a Food Safety Culture.

Fig. 9.2 Differences between traditional food safety management versus behavior-based food safety management

Traditional food safety management has an overly simplistic view of behavior change; behavior-based food safety management understands that behavior change is complex.

Traditional food safety managers place overemphasis on training and inspections in an attempt to change behavior and achieve results. They believe that desired behavior change can be achieved by simply training employees and inspecting processes and conditions against established standards. But as stated so elegantly by B.F. Skinner (1953), *behavior is a difficult subject, not because it is inaccessible, but because it is extremely complex.* While both of these activities (training and inspections) are important, behavior-based food safety managers realize they are not enough to achieve food safety success. They understand the complexity of behavior and, before jumping to an overly simplistic solution; they study and analyze the cause of the performance problem (lack of skill, ineffective work system, lack of motivation, etc) to propose the right solution.

Traditional food safety management is based on linear cause-and-effect thinking; behavior-based food safety management is based on systems thinking.

Traditional food safety management often addresses specific food safety concerns and strategies in isolation or as individual components, not as a whole or complete system. In other words, it approaches food safety with a sort of linear cause-and-effect thinking. Behavior-based food safety management realizes that this sort of linear cause-and-effect thinking is not fully adequate to address complex issues related to an organization's food safety culture or an employee's adherence to food safety practices. Behavior-based food safety management understands that there are numerous factors (physical, organizational, personal) that affect performance and they consider the totality of the numerous activities an organization may conduct and how they are linked together to influence people's thoughts and behaviors.

And last but not least.

Traditional food safety management is focused on developing a food safety program; behavior-based food safety management is focused on creating a food safety culture.

There is a big difference between the two. Traditional food safety management relies on formal authority to accomplish its objectives. Food safety managers get others to follow them or their program because they have authority over them and they are holding them accountable to the rules. Behavior-based food safety managers also use a system of checks and balances, but they use them differently. For example, they use them to observe employee behaviors related to food safety, give feedback and coaching (both positive and negative) based on the results, and provide motivation for continuous improvement. More importantly, behavior-based food safety managers have figured out a way to go beyond accountability. They've figured out a way to get employees at all levels of the organization to do the right things, not because they're being held accountable to them, but because they believe in and are committed to food safety. They create a *food safety culture*.

Chapter 10
Unwrapping – Thoughts on the Future of Food Safety

> *As for the future, your task is not to foresee it, but to enable it.*
> Antoine de Saint-Exupery (French Writer, 1900–1944)

Most books typically end by wrapping-up or summarizing key thoughts and themes presented throughout the book. This would be a fitting way for me to end this book too. However, in contrast (and consistent with the theme of this book), I'm going to end or close this book by doing something a little less traditional. I'm going to end by "unwrapping" with key thoughts on the future of food safety.

You see, as food safety professionals, I do not believe we should be in the business of simply trying to predict the future or anticipate what the future might bring. I believe we should be more proactive. We should shape and influence the future, all in such a way that results in a safer food supply for consumers around the world.

The Way Forward?

Recent high profile outbreaks of foodborne disease in the United States (and elsewhere) have created political and professional pressure for additional food safety controls and management systems. Some say we need a single food safety agency. By them, I'm reminded of a quote by a Greek philosopher named Petronium way back in 210 BC, who said, "We tend to meet any new situation by re-organizing, and a wonderful method it can be for creating the illusion of progress." Reorganization without true change will only give the illusion of progress.

Others claim HACCP is the answer. Although HACCP is a major step in the right direction, it is not the final destination. We have all seen and heard about foodborne outbreaks caused by foods produced in plants alleging to use HACCP. In addition, some of our nation's largest food recalls have been from plants claiming to have HACCP plans in place.

Regardless of what you think the answer might be to advancing food safety, I believe we are at one of those defining moments for our profession. We stand on the brink of an opportunity to accelerate advances as a profession or continue with the more traditional approaches to food safety.

Although I don't think there is any question that in many parts of the food system and world we have made good progress in the battle against foodborne disease, for those of us with a passion for advancing food safety and protecting public health worldwide, we would like to see even more progress made. Despite the fact that thousands of employees have been trained in food safety around the world, millions have been spent globally on food safety research, and countless inspections and tests have been performed at home and abroad, food safety remains a significant public health challenge.

Making Significant Leaps

With this thought in mind, let me share with you what I believe are four critical success factors needed to make significant leaps in food safety.

1. **To make significant leaps in food safety, we need creativity and innovation:** A simple definition of an innovation is the act of introducing something new. From a food safety perspective, an innovation can be a new or enhanced food safety practice, a new food safety product, or a new food production technology. The bottom line is that creativity and innovation leads to change and change can lead to even greater reductions in the risk of food borne disease. Simply put, it is impossible to advance food safety without change.

2. **To make significant leaps in food safety, we need leadership:** As I have shared before, it's interesting to me that in the field of food safety today, we often talk about food safety management. We rarely talk about food safety leadership. But management and leadership are different. According to Stephen Covey, Merrill and Merrill (1994), "Management works within the system; leadership works on the system." Food safety management focuses on the administration of set procedures within an established risk management system; food safety leadership focuses on the creation of new and enhanced risk reduction strategies, models, and processes. In other words, food safety managers deal with planning, directing, and overseeing specific details of the system. Food safety leaders, in contrast, see the need for improvement, create a compelling vision for change, and inspire innovation, all of which lead to even greater reductions in food borne disease. To advance food safety, some of us need to be courageous pioneers and help lead the way.

3. **To make significant leaps in food safety, we need more research:** There is no question about it, we need to be continual learners and more research is needed to answer some of the food safety questions of our day.

   In this era of rapid change, new scientific facts are being discovered at an unprecedented rate. As a food safety professional, are you hanging onto old principles that have been disproved by the latest science? I came across a quote by Dee Hock that summarizes this point quite well. He said, "The problem is never how to get new, innovative thoughts into your mind, but how to get old ones out. Every mind is a room packed with archaic furniture. You must get the old furniture of what you know, think, and believe out before anything new can get in." Also, we need to get better at taking research out of the lab and putting it in contact with the problems in the real world (in a manner that is effective, reliable, and efficient). We also need to learn from other disciplines such as the medical, information technology, and biotechnology fields to name just a few. I believe some of our greatest future food safety solutions may not even come from within the field of food safety.

4. **To make significant leaps in food safety, we need better collaboration:** Remember, the way we get our food from farm to fork, the food system, has become increasingly complex and interdependent on many businesses and individuals. Today more than ever, food safety is truly a shared responsibility. Regulators, academicians, consumers, and industry professionals must recognize that we can do more to advance food safety by working together than by working alone.

The Future

Over the past few years as an executive board member of the International Association for Food Protection, I have been very fortunate to meet many food safety professionals from all over the country and world. It is because of this experience that I remain convinced that the future of food safety looks very bright. Never before in history have we, as a profession, been so well suited to advance food safety through innovation, leadership, research, and collaboration.

Working together, my colleagues and friends, we can make a difference, advance food safety worldwide, and create a *food safety culture* around the world.

Until next time, thanks for reading.

References

Andreasen, A. R. (1995). *Marketing social change: Changing behavior to promote health, social development, and the environment*. San Francisco, California: Jossey-Bass Publishers.

Baranowski, T., Perry, C. L., & Parcel, G. (2002). How individuals, environments, and health behaviors interact: Social cognitive theory. In K. Glanz, F. M. Lewis, & B. K. Rimer, (Eds.), *Health behavior and health education: Theory, research and practice* (3rd ed., pp. 246–279). San Francisco, CA: Jossey-Bass.

Bryan, F. L., Guzewich, J. J., & Todd, E. C. D. (1997). Surveillance of food borne disease I: Purposes and types of surveillance systems and networks. *Journal of Food Protection, 60*, 555–566.

CDC. (2006). Preliminary foodnet data on the incidence of infection with pathogens transmitted commonly through food – 10 States, United States, 2005, *MMWR, 55*(14), 392–395.

CDC. (2007). Preliminary foodnet data on the incidence of infection with pathogens transmitted commonly through food – 10 States, United States, 2006, *MMWR, 56*(14), 336–339.

Cialdini, R. B. (1993). *Influence: The psychology of persuasion*. Revised Edition. New York: William Morrow and Company, Inc.

Cliver, D. O. (1990). *Foodborne diseases*. San Diego, California: Academic Press, Inc.

Columbia Accident Investigation Board. (2003) *Columbia accident investigation report*. Washington, D. C.: Government Printing Office

Coreil, J., Bryant, C. A., & Henderson, J. N. (2001). *Social and behavioral foundations of public health*. Thousand Oaks, California: Sage Publications, Inc.

Covey, S. A., Merrill, R., & Merrill, R.R. (1994). *First things first: To live, to love, to learn, to leave a legacy*. New York: Simon and Schuster.

Daniels, A. C. (1999). *Bringing out the best in people: How to apply the astonishing power of positive reinforcement*. New York, NY: McGraw-Hill.

Daniels, A. C., & Daniels, J. E. (2004). *Performance management: Changing behaviors that drives organizational effectiveness* (4th ed.). Atlanta, GA: Aubrey Daniels International, Inc.

Ebbin, R. (2001). Americans' dining-out habits. *Restaurants USA, 20*, 38–40.

Food and Drug Administration. (2001). *Food code*. Springfield, Virginia: National Technical Information Services.

FDA Retail Food Program Steering Committee. (2000). Report of the FDA Retail Food Program Database of Foodborne Illness Risk Factors. Available via the Internet at http://www.cfsan.fda.gov/~acrobat/retrsk.pdf.

FDA National Retail Food Team. (2004). FDA Report on the Occurrence of Foodborne Illness Risk Factors in Selected Institutional Foodservice, Restaurant, and Retail Food Store Facility Types. Available via the Internet http://www.cfsan.fda.gov/~acrobat/retrsk2.pdf

Fournies, F. F. (1999). *Why employees don't do what they're supposed to do and what to do about it*. Updated Edition. New York: McGraw-Hill.

Gallup. (1999). *Gallup study of changing food preparation and eating habits*. Princeton, NJ: Gallup.

Geller, E. S. (2005). *People-based safety: The source*. Virginia Beach, Virginia: Coastal.

Gostick, A., & Elton, C. (2007). *The carrot principle: How the best managers use recognition to engage their people, retain talent, and accelerate performance*. New York, NY: Free Press.

Health and Safety Commission. (1993). Third report of the Advisory Committee on the Safety of Nuclear Installations: Organising for Safety. ISBN 0-11-882104-0.

Hedberg, C. W., Smith, S. J., Kirkland, E., Radke, V., Jones, T. F., Selman, A. S., et al. (2006). Systematic environmental evaluations to identify food safety differences between outbreak and nonoutbreak restaurants. *Journal of Food Protection, 69*, 2697–2702.

Janz, N. K., Champion, V. L., & Strecher, V. J. (2002). The health belief model. In K. Glanz, F. M. Lewis, & B. K. Rimer, (Eds.), *Health behavior and health education: Theory, research, and practice* (3rd ed., pp. 45–66). San Francisco, CA: Jossey-Bass.

Jones, T. F., Pavlin, B. I., LaFleur, B. J., Ingram, L. A., & Schaffner, W. (2004). Restaurant inspection scores and food borne diseases. *Emerging Infectious Diseases, 10*, 668–692.

LeBoeuf, M. (1985). *The greatest management principle in the world*. New York: Putnam.

Leeds, D. (2000). *The 7 powers of questions: Secrets to successful communication in life and at work*. New York: Penguin Putnam, Inc.

Madesen, C. H., Jr., & Madsen, C. R. (1974). *Teaching and discipline: Behavior principles toward a positive approach*. Boston: Allyn & Bacon.

Maxwell, J. C. (1998). *The 21 irrefutable laws of leadership: Follow them and people will follow you*. Nashville, Tennessee: Thomas Nelson, Inc.

Mead, P. S., Slutsker, L., Dietz, V., et al. (1999). Food-related illness and death in the United States. *Emerging Infectious Diseases, 5*, 607–625.

Montano, D. E., & Kasprzyk, D. (2002). The theory of reasoned action and the theory of planned behavior. In K. Glanz, F. M. Lewis, & B. K. Rimer (Eds.), *Health behavior and health education: Theory, research and practice* (3rd ed., pp. 85–112). San Francisco, CA: Jossey-Bass.

Mullen, L. A., Cowden, J. M., Cowden, D., & Wong, R. (2002). An evaluation of the risk assessment method used by environmental health officers when inspecting food businesses. *International Journal of Environmental Health Research, 12*, 255–260.

NRA. (2001). Industry at a glance. National Restaurant Association. Available via the Internet at http://www.restaurant.org/research/ind_glance.cfm

NRA. (2006). State of the restaurant industry workforce: an overview. National Restaurant Association. Available via the Internet at http://www.restaurant.org/pdfs/research/workforce_overview.pdf

Olsen, S. J., MacKinon, L. C., Goulding, J. S., Bean, N. H., & Slutsker, L. (2000). Surveillance for food borne disease outbreaks – United States. 1993–1997. *MMWR 49* (SS01), 1–51.

OSHA. (1996). Presenting effective presentation with visual aids. Construction OSHA Office of Training and Education. Available via the Internet at www.osha-slc.gov/doc/outreach training/htmlfiles/traintec.html

OSHA. (1998). Training Requirements in OSHA Standards and Training Guidelines. Available via the Internet at www.osha.gov/Publications/osha2254.pdf.

Prichard, R. D., Jones, S. D., & Roth, P. L. (1988). Effects of group feedback, goal setting, and incentives on organizational productivity. *Journal of Applied Psychology, 73*, 337–358.

Prochaska, J. O., & DiClemente, C. C. (1986). Toward a comprehensive model of change. In W. R. Miller & N. Heather (Eds,), *Treating addictive behaviors: Process of change. Applied clinical psychology* (pp 3–27). New York: Plenum.

Redmond, E. C., & Griffith, C. J. (2006). Assessment of consumer food safety education provided by local authorities in the UK. *British Food Journal, 108*(9), pp 732–751.

Schein, E. (1992). Organizational Culture and Leadership, 2nd Ed. San Francisco, California: Jossey-Bass.

References

Sertkaya, A., Berlind, A. Lange, R., & Zink, D. (2006). Top ten food safety problems in the United States food processing industry. *Food Protection Trends, 26*(5), 310–315.

Skinner, B. F. (1953). *Science and human behavior*. New York: Macmillan.

Slovic, P. (1991). Beyond numbers: A broader perspective on the risk perception and risk communication. In D. G. Mayo & R. D. Hollander (Eds.), *Acceptable evidence: Science and values in risk management*(pp. 48–65). New York: Oxford University Press.

United States Department of Agriculture. (2006). Progress Report on Salmonella Testing of Raw Meat and Poultry Products, 1998–2005. Available via the internet at http://www.fsis.usda.gov/science/progress_ report_salmonella_testing/index.asp

United States Department of Agriculture, Economic Research Service. 2006. Food Market Structures. Available via the internet at http://www.ers.usda.gov/Briefing/FoodMarket Structures/

Whiting, M. A., & Bennett, C. J. (2003). *Driving toward "O": Best practices in corporate safety and health*. The Conference Board. Research Report R-1334-03-RR

Index

Note: The letter *f* in the index refers to figures, for example 64*f* refers to figure in page 64

A
Accident investigation root causes, 13*f*
Andreasen, A. R., 25

B
Baranowski, T., 23–24
Bean, N. H., 4
Behavior, education and training, 39–45
    See also Educating and training to influence behavior
Behavioral theory
    operant conditioning, 23
Behavior-based food safety management, 77–81
    management/leadership, differences, 77–78
    systems
        consequences, 67–74
        continuous improvement model, 27*f*, 78*f*
        See also Consequences, increase/decrease behaviors
    traditional *vs.* behavior-based food, 78–81
Behavior-based food safety managers, 79–80
Behavior change theories and model
    behavioral theory, 23
        operant conditioning, 23
    health belief model, 24
    social cognitive theory, 23–24
        central concepts, 24
        concepts, self-efficacy/skills, 24
    social marketing, 25
    theory of reasoned action, 24
    transtheoretical model, 24–25
Bennett, C. J., 15, 17
Berlind, A., 39
Bryan, F. L., 11, 33
Bryant, C. A., 11

C
Campylobacter, 7
CCP, *see* Critical control points (CCP)
Centers for Disease Control and Prevention, 4, 25
    risk factors, foodborne diseases, 33
Champion, V. L., 24
Cialdini, R. B., 15
Cliver, D. O., 3
Communicating food safety
    conversations, importance of, 52–53
    food safety culture survey questionnaire, 55*f*
    importance of, 49–50
    with individuals, non-English speaking, 52
    medium, variety of, 50
    posters/symbols/slogans, 51
        tips on making, 51
    questions, importance of asking, 54
    visualization, effect of, 51–52
Consequences, increase/decrease behaviors
    creation of, 69–70
    effects of, 69*f*
    negative consequences, 73–74
    performance problems, cause of, 68–69
    positive consequences, 70–73
Coreil, J., 11
Covey, S. A., 84
Cowden, D., 6
Cowden, J. M., 6
Critical control points (CCP), 7
Culture, 11–18
    best practices, 17–18
    core elements
        accountability, 17
        confidence in employees, 16
        knowledge sharing and information, 17

Culture (*cont.*)
  leadership, 16
    management visibility and
      leadership, 16
  creation of, 13–15
    intentional commitment/hard
      work, 15
  definition, 11–12
  foundation, 15
  importance of, 12–13

D
Daniels, A. C., 58, 67
Daniels, J. E., 58
Developing food safety goals
    and measurements
  effective food safety goals,
    establishment, 58–59
    important things, 58–59
  goal setting, importance of, 57–58
  leading *vs.*lagging indicators of food
    safety, 62–65, 64*f*
  measurements, maximize use of,
    59–61
  process/knowledge/behavior,
    measurement of, 61–62
DiClemente, C. C., 24
Dietz, V., 4
*Driving Towards "0", Best Practices in
    Corporate Safety and Health, How
    Leading Companies Develop Safety
    Cultures,*15

E
Ebbin, R., 3
Educating and training to influence
    behavior, 39–45
  diversity, value/respect, 44–45
    native language, education in, 45
  education *vs.*training, 40–41
  focus on changing behavior, 42–44
  process of, 46
  reason, education and training, 41
  risk-based, 44
  simple and user friendly, 45–46
Elton, C., 71
Employees, dealing with
    gastrointestinal symptoms, with, 34
Environmental Health Services, 25
Estimate of food allergic consumers/
    reactions in United States, 42*f*
Estimate of foodborne disease in the United
    States per year, 5*f*

F
FDA baseline surveys, suggestions, 6
FDA food code table of contents (2001), 32*f*
Food allergy, 35
  employees behavior towards, 35
  estimate of food allergic consumers/
    reactions in United States, 42*f*
  Sarah Weaver story, 44*f*–45*f*
Food and Drug Administration
  Food Code, 26
  purpose, 32
Foodborne disease, 4–6
  outbreaks, factors of, 8, 8*f*
  restaurant-associated, 6
  surveillance, 63
Foodborne outbreaks in United States
  by contributing factor (CDC,
    1993–1997), 33*f*
  by place, reports, 5*f*
Food production
  food safety awareness, 1
  history of, 1–3
  retail food establishments,
    emergence of, 3–4
  retail food safety
    changing behavior, 8–9
    reducing risk in food production
      chain, 6–8
Food safety
  communication plan, *see*
    Communicating food safety
  conversations, importance of, 53
  culture-not a food safety program, 12*f*
  culture survey questionnaire, 55*f*
  education, 40–41
  education/training, tips for designing, 42
  educator, 45–46, 54
  effective communication,
    see Communicating food safety
  equation, 2*f*
  future, success factors
    collaboration, better, 85
    creativity and innovation, 84
    leadership, 84
    research, more of, 84–85
  goals measurement development,
    see Developing food safety goals
    and measurements
  lagging *vs.*leading indicators of,
    62–65
  management system, behavior- based,
    9, 21–22, 28, 29, 36, 39, 46, 54,
    57, 65, 74, 77–79

factors (physical, organizational, personal), 80
professionals, 18, 21–22, 29, 39, 42, 45, 50, 54, 59, 62, 70, 83, 85
smart questions, 54
systems-based approach, 21–28
See also Systems-based approach to food safety
training, 41
Food safety performance expectations, creation of
beyond regulatory compliance, 34–35
develop risk-based expectations, 32–34
gastrointestinal symptoms, employees with, 34
temperature, suitable/ refrigeration, 34
documentation of, 35–36
efficiency, 30
employees, work of, 29–30
FDA food code table of contents (2001), 32*f*
food code, 32
guiding principles, 35–36, 36*f*
proper food safety attitude, 31
specific behaviors related to risk factors, 34*f*
specificity, 31–32
phrases/fancy slogans, 32
Food safety system, 26*f*
3 A Systems-Based Approach, 25*f*
Food sciences, understanding of, 9
Food security, 35
Fournies, F. F., 29, 68
Future of food safety, success factors
collaboration, better, 85
creativity and innovation, 84
leadership, 84
research, more of, 84–85

G
Gallup, G., 3
Gastrointestinal illnesses, 4
Geller, E. S., 14, 15, 25
GMPs, *see* Good manufacturing practices (GMPs)
Good manufacturing practices (GMPs), 21, 79
Gostick, A., 71

Goulding, J. S., 4
The Greatest Management Principle in the World, 73
Griffith, C. J., 6, 50
Guzewich, J. J., 33

H
HACCP, *see* Hazard Analysis and Critical Control Point (HACCP)
Hazard Analysis and Critical Control Point (HACCP), 17, 55, 60, 64, 72, 83
Health and Safety Commission (1993) safety culture, technical definition, 12
Health belief model, 24
Hedberg, C. W., 62
Henderson, J. N., 11
History of food production foodborne disease, 1–3

I
Influence, The Psychology of Persuasion, 15
Ingram, L. A., 6
International Association for Food Protection, 85
International Food Safety Icons (IAFP), 52, 53*f*

J
Janz, N. K., 24
Jones, S. D., 58
Jones, T. F., 6, 61

K
Kasprzyk, D., 24

L
LaFleur, B. J., 6
Lange, R., 39
LeBoeuf, M., 73
Leeds, D., 54

M
MacKinon, L. C., 4
Madsen, C. R., 71
Management-created consequences, 70
Maxwell, J. C., 16
Mead, P. S., 4
Merrill, R. R., 84
Modern food system, interdependency, 2
Montano, D. E., 24
Mullen, L. A., 6, 61

N

National Center for Environmental Health, 25
Native language, importance, 45
Negative consequences, food safety management, 73–74

O

Occupational Safety and Health Administration's Training Guideline (OSHA), 39
Occupational safety and health administration's training model (1998), 40*f*
Olsen, S. J., 4, 8, 33, 44
Operant conditioning, 23
 See also Behavior change theories and model
Organization
 culture, influence of, 13
 safety culture of, 12
  characteristics, 12
 values or beliefs, 15
 violations per inspection, 31
 zero-tolerance philosophy, 31
OSHA, *see* Occupational Safety and Health Administration's Training Guideline (OSHA)

P

Parcel, G., 23–24
Pavlin, B. I., 6
Perception, individual, 24
 See also Health belief model
Performance problems
 ineffective system, 68
 motivation, lack of, 69
 skill, lack of, 68
 See also Consequences, increase/decrease behaviors
Perry, C. L., 23–24
Personal testimonials, 42–43
Positive and negative consequences on behavior, effects of, 69*f*
Positive consequences, food safety performance
 outcomes, 72–73
 process/conditions, 72
 specific desired behaviors, 71–72
Positive/negative reinforcement, 69
Positive safety culture, organizations with

The 7 Powers of Questions: Secrets to Successful Communication in Life and at Work, 54
Prochaska, J. O., 24
Public health professionals
 health belief model, 24
 See also Behavior change theories and model
Punishment and penalty, 69

R

Ranking of food safety problems by number of votes across all sectors, 40*f*
Ready-to-eat meals, 4
Redmond, E. C., 50
Reinforcement
 positive/negative, 69
 and recognition, 71
Restaurant employees speaking language other than English at home, 4*f*
Retail food establishments
 emergence of, 3–4
 employees speaking language other than English at home, 4*f*
 restaurant industry, United States, 3
 supermarkets, 3
 hand washing facility, 26
 outer openings, 26
 restaurant industry, 3
Retail food safety
 changing behavior, 8–9
 food sciences, understanding of, 9
 primary methods, reduce risk of disease, 6, 9
 reducing risk in food production chain, 6–8
  CCP, 7
  pathogenic organisms, eliminating, 7
  SCP, visual model, 7*f*
 regulatory inspections, 6, 9
 training, 6, 9
Roth, P. L., 58

S

Safety culture
 best practices, 18*f*
 in organization, 12
Sarah Weaver story, 43*f*–44*f*
Schaffner, W., 6
SCP, *see* Strategic control point (SCP)
Self-efficacy, 24
 See also Behavior change theories and model

Sertkaya, A., 39, 40
Skinner, B. F., 23, 67, 80
Slovic, P., 42
Slutsker, L., 4
Social cognitive theory, 23–24
Social marketing, 25
Soft stuff, 11
Specific behaviors related to risk factors, 34f
Standardized drawings, tools for communication, 52
Strategic control point (SCP) visual model, 7
Supermarkets, 3
Systems-based approach to food safety, 21–28
 behavior-based systems continuous improvement model, 27–28
 behavior change theories and model
  behavioral theory, 23
  health belief model, 24
  social cognitive theory, 23–24
  social marketing, 25
  theory of reasoned action, 24
  transtheoretical model, 24–25
 definition, 22
 environmental/physical factors, 25–27
 systems thinking, 22–23
Systems thinking
 simple linear cause and effect relationship, 23f
 simple system feedback relationship, 23f

T
Theory of reasoned action, 24
 See also Behavior change theories and model
Todd, E. C. D., 33
Tools, enhance food safety performance, 70
Traditional food safety managers, 79–80
Traditional *vs.* behavior-based food safety management, differences, 78–81, 79f
Transtheoretical model
 stages, 24–25
 See also Behavior change theories and model

U
United States Department of Agriculture, Economic Research Service (2006) food system, definition, 2

V
Visual aids, food safety, 52, 53f
Visualization, communication through, 52

W
Whiting, M. A., 15, 17
Wong, R., 6

Z
Zink, D., 39

Printed in the United States of America

PRESTON COLLEGE
LIBRARY LEARNING CENTRES